CHAKRA HEALING FOR BEGINNERS

A COMPLETE GUIDE TO BALANCE CHAKRA THROUGH MEDITATION TO HEAL YOUR BODY AND INCREASE POSITIVE ENERGY INCLUDES SECRET TIPS FOR THIRD EYE AWAKENING

ISBN: 9798630043788

Contents

Introduction

The history of the Chakras is one that is rich with different opinions and various origins. Many religious and spiritual belief systems contain information that relates to the Chakra system, but each has its own words, terminology, and overarching rules. What remains the same, however, is the basic understanding that contained within the body is a powerful energy that can have a wide range of effects on our mental, physical, and spiritual health.

Regardless of your own personal religious or spiritual background, the knowledge of the Chakras can have a positive impact on your own life, making it very worthwhile to take the time to understand. But before we dive into why the Chakras are so integral, we must first begin with what exactly they are.

The Meaning behind the Chakras

The word Chakra is derived from an Indian word "Chakra" which literally translates to mean "wheel". Each Chakra can be visualized as a spinning wheel within the body that houses the energy of that particular system. In total, there are seven distinct Chakras, each controlling and maintaining a certain part of the body, as well as different qualities within us. The Chakras are both located within the physical body, as well as being a mental and spiritual focal point for us to use within meditation and other energy healing rituals.

Many of us understand that the mind and bodywork in tandem, affecting one another and influencing how each functions. But, few of us truly understand the difference between the physical body and the mental energy that sounds it, and how those two systems are integral to one another. In all traditions that incorporate the knowledge of the Chakras, it is accepted that there is an energy that surrounds and runs through the body. This energy is commonly referred to as the "subtle body", a term that helps differentiate the physical experience from the spiritual one. The subtle body corresponds to a plane of existence that is outside of the physical realm in which we exist. This plane is connected to a higher concept, a higher realm of existence, and is spiritual rather than physical.

The concepts of the subtle body and various planes of existence can be extremely complicated and difficult to understand, so to avoid confusion we will focus just on the Chakras and how they impact the physical experience of all of us.

While we cannot actually see the Chakras, their influence in our lives can be felt daily. In total, there are seven different Chakras, which form a line from the foot of our spine up to the top of our head. Some religious belief systems disagree about how many Chakras there are, with some saying there are only five, and others saying there are thousands, but the most common understanding accepts the standard seven.

Each Chakra, as you can see, corresponds to a particular area of the body and it has a great impact on each of those systems. When the Chakras are closed off or unbalanced, they can result in physical ailments and other problems which can negatively impact our lives. In order to have a healthy and functioning mental and physical experience, it is encouraged that each person learns how to open each Chakra and keep them balanced and circulating.

Now, you may be asking yourself what exactly is meant when we talk about opening or balancing your Chakras. If you are struggling in your personal relationships, have difficulty sleeping, feel anxious, or get sick easily, then you may have an imbalance in your Chakras that are helping to cause these problems. If you can focus on each of the Chakras, you can identify where you are stuck and the underlying cause that is creating the imbalance. From here, through various exercises and techniques, you can fix the issue so that your energy flows properly once more.

Origins of the Chakra System

The Chakra system can be traced back many centuries, with the first usage of the term Chakras being seen in the Hindu Vedas. Written in ancient India, the Vedas are some of the oldest religious texts in existence and can be dated back to around the 1st and 2nd century BCE.

Chapter 1.
Identifying Chakras

'Chakra' is a Sanskrit word meaning wheel. The earliest recorded mention of the Chakras is at least 5000 years old. Hindu scriptures, called the 'Vedas,' have an elaborate description of the chakra system and the role it plays in our lives. The Buddhist and Jain scriptures also have the mention of the chakra system. Chakras are not a new discovery or gimmick. The power of chakras had been discovered thousands of years ago, and people made use of that knowledge to remain healthy and happy even when modern medical science was not at their disposal. Understanding of the chakras can help you in discovering some interesting things about health and life.

We all have a physical body that can be seen, touched, and felt. It consists of an elaborate system of blood, bones, muscles, nerves, and the works. However, besides the physical body, there is also an energy body. It consists of the energy that flows inside us. It keeps us powered and makes the system work.

Our body is a big bundle of energy. There is a constant energy transfer going on. Every part of the body needs energy. However, the needs of every part are different. All the body parts do not need energy at the same rate or quantity. The role of the chakras is to regulate this flow and ensure that you achieve your maximum potential.

The chakras are the energy centers. They are the points at which the concentration of this energy is at its peak. These chakras are constantly transferring energy to various parts of the body. The complete system of health and well-being relies heavily upon the functioning of these chakras. If the chakras work in tandem, you will remain healthy and joyful. They will have a profound impact on your physical, mental, emotional, and spiritual well-being.

The Vedas state that there are 144 major and minor chakras in our body. Out of these, there are two chakras that don't need your attention. The remaining 142 chakras play a very active role in ensuring your physical, mental, emotional, and spiritual health.

The chakras are strategically located at the junction points of our nervous system. They ensure a smooth transfer of energy.

These chakras are further divided into seven major chakras that would determine your personality, strengths, and weaknesses. Various factors related to your physical and mental health are also regulated by these chakras.

All seven major chakras are located along your spine. These chakras do not have a physical presence, as they are simply energy points. However, their location on your spine does have a significant impact on the organs in those areas. By keeping your chakras balanced, you can ensure that your vital organs keep working smoothly.

Chakras are constantly spinning energy wheels. Every chakra transfers energy to the other, and this process carries on until the seventh chakra. The higher you go up the chakra scale, the level of intensity it brings into your life would increase. It means if a lower chakra in your body is dominant, it will empower your abilities to feel the worldly pleasures more intensely. You will be able to enjoy the bounties of nature in a better way, as the lower three chakras relate to physical needs, whereas the upper three chakras cater to intellectual needs. If any of the upper three chakras is dominant in your body, you will have a greater affinity toward intellectual and spiritual realization. The higher the chakra, the greater will be the intensity with which it affects your life.

Each chakra has its important characteristics. Whichever chakra becomes dominant in you will give you its traits. It means that your personality is a very good reflection of the most powerful chakra in your body.

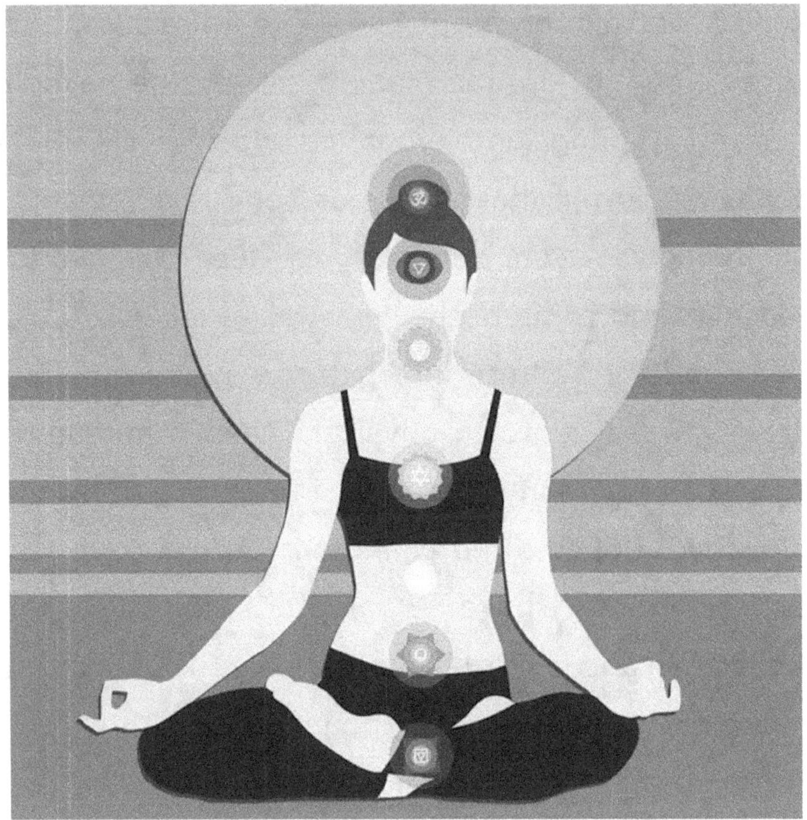

The seven main chakras in our body are the following.

The Root Chakra (Muladhara)

This is the first chakra in our body. It is located at the base of the spine. The most important role of this chakra is to provide you survival instincts. If this chakra is more powerful in your body, basic things like food and sleep will be the most important in your life. These two things may seem to be simple or trivial needs, but if you think deeply, the biggest part of our life revolves around only these two things. All the money we earn and the material wealth we gain is focused on survival and security. Food represents survival, and sleep represents security. This chakra keeps you centered in reality. You feel grounded and connected with basic human nature. Although this is the base chakra, it doesn't mean it is any less important. In fact, even if you seek the realization of the top chakra, proper functioning of the root chakra is of utmost importance. This is the chakra that will help you in remaining focused on reality while you strive for spiritual awakening.

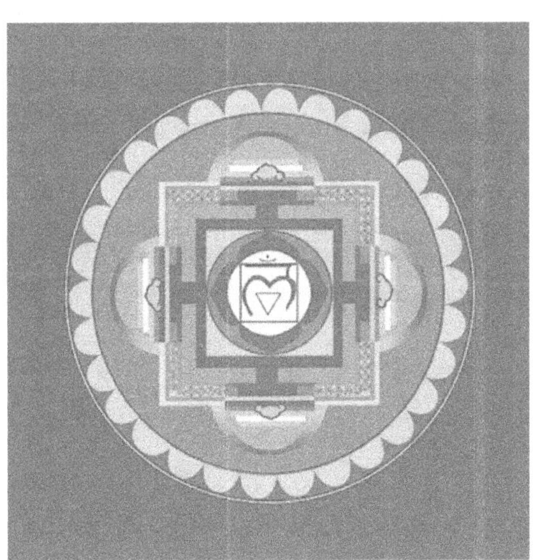

The Sacral Chakra (Svadishthana)

This is the pleasure seeker's chakra. Located approximately two inches below the navel, this chakra gives you the gift to enjoy this world. If this chakra becomes powerful in your body, you will be able to relish all the physical pleasures of this world. Most of the people in this world are unfortunate as they live in the most scenic places but never find them beautiful. Some people can cook the most tasteful delicacies but may not enjoy eating them. A person with power in this chakra will not be among them. A person with power in the sacral chakra will be able to enjoy even the most mundane activities in life. Such a person would have an eye to find joy even in the most inanimate objects. Power in this chakra enables you to live a joyful life. You wouldn't treat life as another passing affair as most of us do. For you, life will be a grand event, and you will have a big role in the grand scheme of things.

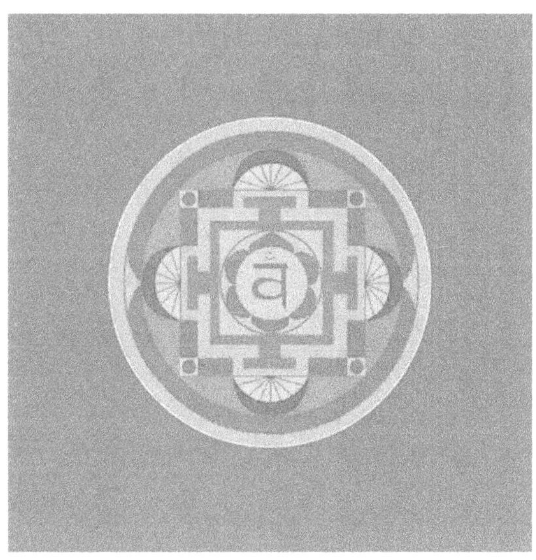

Solar Plexus Chakra (Manipura)

This is the doer's chakra, physically located around two inches above the navel. If this chakra finds expression in your body, it will give you indomitable will and the ability to make your dreams come true. It will make you enterprising. You will become a person who would enjoy working tirelessly. This chakra makes people efficient, hardworking, and zealous. Whether it is the field of politics, education, science, or commerce, this chakra can make you shine in every field. A person with this chakra in dominance would not understand the vice of procrastination. You'd never be able to leave work for tomorrow. 'If something can be done today, it must be done immediately' would be your life mantra. This chakra can make you intense and deeply focused.

The Heart Chakra (Anahata)

This chakra is located in the center of your chest. The meaning of this chakra is the unstruck sound, which means the energy of this chakra knows no bounds. It is boundless and ever-expanding. This is the center chakra in your body. Out of the seven chakras, this is the chakra that comes between the top and bottom three chakras. It is equidistant from the chakras that increase your attachment to the body and also from the chakras that increase your affinity toward intellectuality and spirituality. This is the chakra that helps you in finding a middle ground. It enables you to be creative. This means that you can find intellectual and spiritual meaning in the physical things of this world. This chakra can change the way you look at this world. It makes you more sensitive, emotional, generous, and empathetic. If this chakra is more powerful in your body, you will be able to feel the pain of the most impassive things in this world and express them with greater intensity. It makes you a creative person by nature. This is the fourth chakra in your body. Hence, the intensity of this chakra is higher than those preceding it. If it is a pain of others, you will be able to feel it very deeply. You may get disturbed when looking at others in pain. Tears may well up in your eyes whenever you deal with something emotional. You will live life much more intentionally than others.

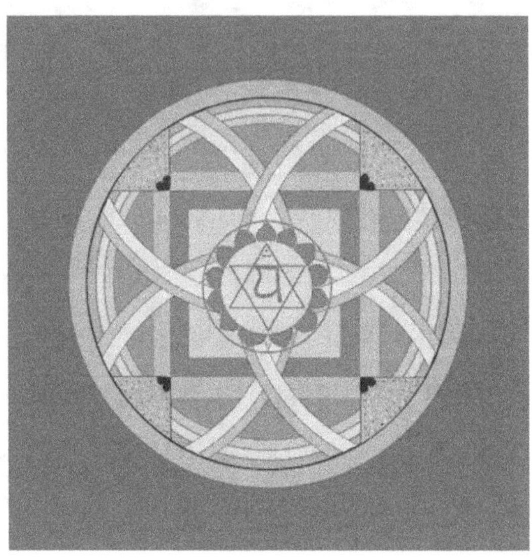

The Throat Chakra (Vishuddhi)

This is the fifth chakra in the sequence, located in front of the base of your neck. The hollow point in the center of your collar bones is the exact location of this chakra. This is the chakra that makes you immensely powerful. This chakra will empower you with the gift of expression and communication. People with powerful throat chakra can hold the masses with their gaze. They command undisputed authority and popularity. This is the chakra of the skilled and crafty people. It empowers you to master your craft with excellence. You get learning abilities like no one else in your genre. This is the chakra that can produce leaders of the masses. These are people with an amazing gift of words. Even your presence would speak volumes about your power in the room.

This is one of the most powerful chakras in the body. The power of this chakra resides in the fact that this chakra can also give you metaphysical powers. This may look like an exaggeration to a beginner, but it is an established fact that power in this chakra can increase your sense of perception. This means that you will be able to feel things that others can't. You will be able to feel not only tangible things in this world but also the intangible ones. Your perception of things increases energy levels. It means you will be able to feel the presence of different kinds of energies around you. It may also empower you to harness these energies for various chores. If you want to enhance your psychic abilities, then this is also the chakra you should be working on. If the third eye chakra is active in you, your psychic abilities will improve tremendously.

The third eye is the second chakra from the top, and it is highly focused on spiritual consciousness. This means the power in this chakra will help your understanding of spiritual matters.

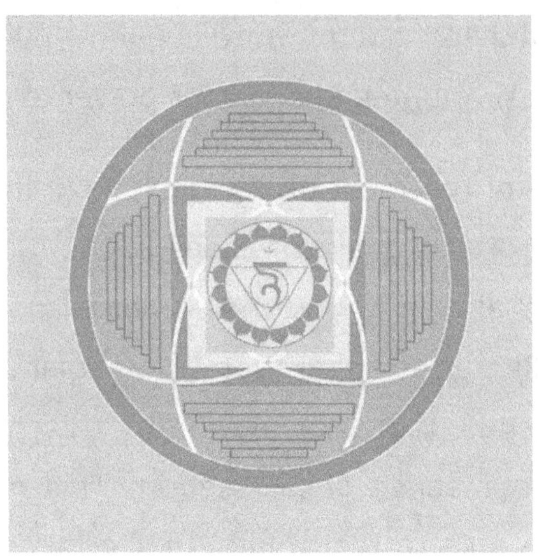

Third Eye Chakra (Ajna)

This is the sixth chakra and is called the third eye chakra. It is located in the middle of the forehead, between the eyebrows. This is a very spiritual chakra and is connected to the metaphysical world. It helps you connect to your higher self, and develop and nurture psychic abilities such as telepathy, astral travel, scrying, sensing events yet to happen, and connecting to past lives. The third eye is also an especially strong link between the spiritual and physical strength. A balanced third eye chakra can help improve your intuition and mental and spiritual clarity, strengthen your faith, make it easier for you to receive and accept spiritual guidance, and understand yourself on a much higher level. It can also encourage you to become more selfless, and increase your potential to develop psychic skills more easily and at a faster rate.

The third eye chakra is connected to the eyes, pituitary gland, endocrine system, and brain. Typical physical manifestations of an imbalanced third eye chakra are eye-related problems such as blurry vision or pain, sleeping disorders, headaches or migraines, and learning disabilities.

The third eye crystal is linked to the color indigo and the element of light. It is depicted by a two-petaled lotus.

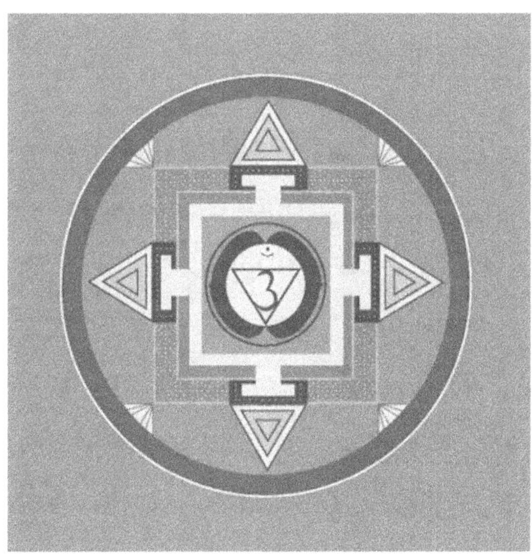

The Crown Chakra (Sahasrara)

This is the seventh chakra, and it is located at the top of your head. The physical location of this chakra is not inside your body but exactly on top of it. This is the chakra you should be working on if spiritual consciousness is your goal. If this chakra is powerful in your body, you will find this world to be very small for yourself. You will be full of energy and have the abilities to look beyond the visible things. This chakra gives you several abilities for you to feel more intellectually and spiritually realized. If this chakra becomes powerful, your physical aspirations diminish, and your spiritual hunger gets stronger. You will be the person who can ponder over the big questions of life and enlighten the world with pure knowledge.

These seven chakras hold the key to human consciousness. They regulate and influence our behavior. They have the ability to make us feel good, as well as pathetic. If your chakras are balanced and in harmony with each other, you may feel blessed even with limited means. However, if some of your chakras are blocked or out of sync, you may feel pathetic, even with all the material wealth at your disposal. They have everything they need, yet they feel a big void inside them. They keep looking for that one thing, which can make them feel complete but never find it. The reason for their failure is their misdirection. They are looking for a solution outside, while the problem is inside.

Ideally, the chakras should be active and balanced. However, the chakras function on a delicate balance of energy. This is heavily influenced by the kind of food you eat, your lifestyle, and your physical and emotional state as well. It is not very uncommon to have an imbalance in the chakras. Some chakras in the body can start functioning hyperactively. This happens when your inclination toward a particular thing grows very strongly. A chakra can start under-functioning when you start avoiding a particular thing or trait associated with that chakra. All such things keep happening inside the body, as energy is always in motion. However, if a chakra remains imbalanced, blocked, or hyperactive for very long, it can affect the functioning of your other chakras, too. Remember, all chakras are connected to each other. So, if one chakra is not working properly, it would affect the flow of energy in the body. The physical organs influenced by that chakra would also get affected.

Therefore, it is very important that you clearly understand the impact of chakras on your body and the influence they can have if there is an imbalance in the chakras. This will help you in preventing problems in life.

This book will help you in understanding chakras and the profound impact the chakras have on your character, personality, behavior, and functioning. You will get to know the ways in which imbalance in chakras can create havoc in your life and the techniques to balance the chakras.

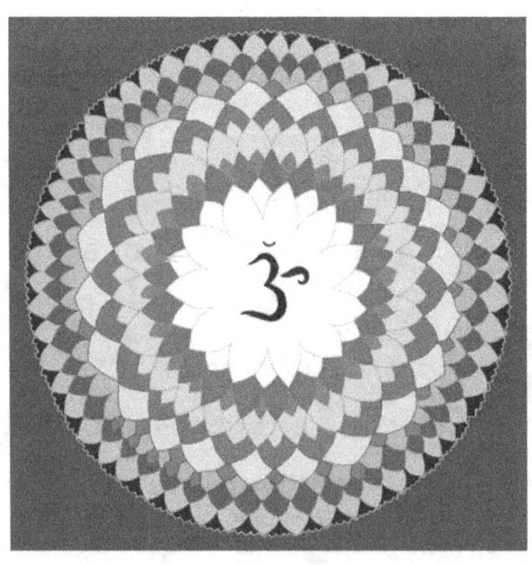

Chapter 2.
Chakra Meditation

Choosing a Meditation

Before deciding which meditation you want to practice, you'll first need to determine which chakras you'll focus your energy on, which chakra to start with, and in which order to address the other chakras. You'll also want to evaluate the timeframe you have to work with for the day and then set aside time in your schedule for meditation.

ONE CHAKRA OR MANY?

The order won't negatively affect any of your other chakras. However, a good general rule is to work on the chakra with the most issues first. I recommend that you listen to your intuition to determine which chakra is giving you the most trouble.

Some chakra experts prefer to work from the center out, because the central chakras—heart and solar plexus—tend to become "stuck" due to their locations. Another option is to start with the root space and then move up to the crown. Opening these end chakras usually will bring about a big shift, so your energy can flow and balance can naturally return.

I prefer to work on the heart chakra first because this chakra is the ultimate connection to your infinite being. I usually find that once the heart chakra is cleared, energy issues within other chakras are easier to resolve. For example, say I am experiencing emotional pain from a breakup, and because I have not dealt with those feelings, I am also experiencing anxiety and back pain. My solar plexus is being affected as well as my heart space. I would first want to focus on heart-based healing and then on my solar plexus to address my physical symptoms.

TIME AS A FACTOR

The meditations in this book fit into 5-, 15-, or 30-minute time-frames to make finding a meditation that will suit your schedule easy. The five-minute meditations are a nice way to dip your toes in the water before you get into the deep end. They are also perfect for energetic maintenance. The longer meditations will help you unlock your creativity and examine personal connections in deep and profound ways. They will yield great insights, clarity, and focus and make your practice more meaningful.

To really clear a chakra on your own, without Reiki or the use of other energy modalities, you'll want to sit with that specific chakra for a minimum of 30 to 45 minutes. You'll have the option to extend all of the meditations in this book with additional breathing and visualization exercises. Time is of the essence, so choose your meditation wisely and commit to it for the minimum suggested length to receive the full benefits.

WHAT'S YOUR INTENTION?

Setting an intention before you begin meditating is the perfect way to formalize what you want to achieve. An intention also improves your odds of successfully making your wish a reality. For example, you may want to achieve balance. Maybe you want a more harmonious relationship with yourself or another person. Perhaps you have an urgent health issue. Maybe you're tackling a bigger issue, such as what you want most out of your life.

Whatever your need, just remember that a restorative or preventative long-term practice will look and feel different than a practice that directly addresses an immediate need, such as a health crisis. Be sure to check in with yourself before you start each meditation in order to determine your goals. If your intention shifts once you get started, simply adjust. Being open and flexible is how all seasoned meditators achieve the greatest results.

The Elements of Guided Meditation

There are many ways to explore your meditation practice, including mantras, visualizations, breath work, and reflections. You may find it beneficial to begin by practicing a few meditations with a friend. You may also find it beneficial to record yourself reading the meditation instructions so you can play them back whenever you need a reminder.

If you feel called to make one of the mantras the focus of your meditation, you could potentially do a full sit with that mantra and challenge yourself with a timer. You don't have to pair any meditation elements in order for a meditation to be coherent and successful. Once you learn the foundational elements of meditation, you can put them together however you see fit. The beauty of this practice is that it is yours.

MANTRAS AND MUDRA

In Sanskrit, the word mantra can be broken into two parts: man, which means "mind," and tra, which means "vehicle." Therefore, a mantra is essentially a vehicle of the mind, a type of spiritual formula used to quickly take you into a deep state of meditation.

Mantras help you alter your state of consciousness. Chanting a powerful word or phrase, every syllable of which is specifically designed to affect subconscious impulses and habits, helps you transcend thought and heighten your awareness.

Mudras are hand postures or gestures that are practiced with your fingers, and their origins are rooted in Hinduism and Buddhism. Because your hand is mapped to your brain, mudras target the reflex points important for unlocking certain biological signals such as relaxation, metabolic rate, or circulation. Adding mudras to your meditations is not necessary but can complement and enhance your practice.

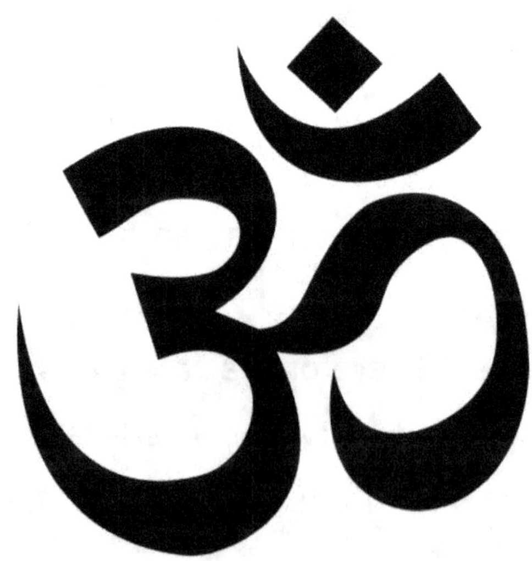

The symbol of Oṃ, the most sacred Hindu mantra

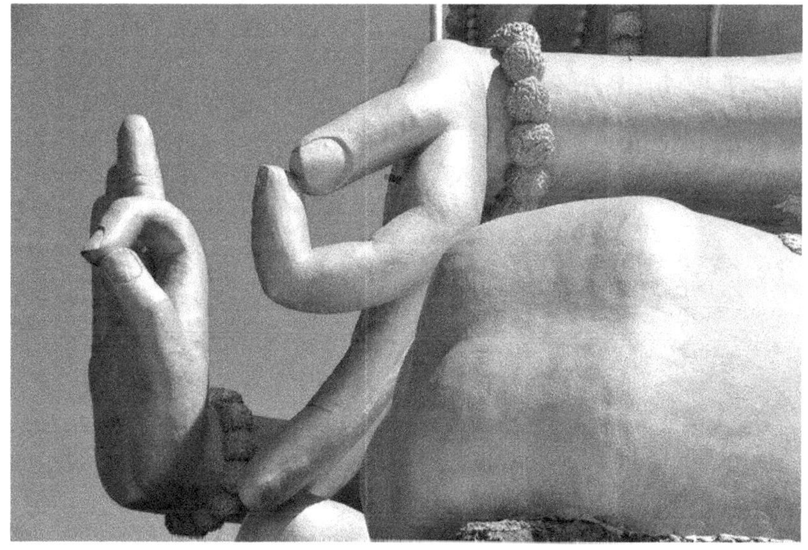

The hands form the Dhyanamudra

VISUALIZATION

Many meditations in this book include some type of visualization. Some visualizations involve specific colors or ask you to use your imagination to enhance your experience. But the emphasis should always be on the feeling that the visualization evokes.

Visualization is a powerful meditation tool that's used to influence the physical body as well as desired outcomes, particularly when those outcomes involve health. Deepak Chopra teaches whatever the focus of our attention, it grows stronger; whatever we withdraw our attention from diminishes. Therefore, visualizing wellness creates more of it.

Visualizations are known to manifest specific results with startling accuracy. Creating a mental image of desired feelings and situations helps you elicit them. Use this practice to live in ways that support your desired goals.

Everything is created twice. First in the mind, and then in reality.

—ROBIN S. SHARMA

MEDITATION

For each chakra, I'll guide you through meditations that are 5, 15, and 30 minutes in length and that instruct you to link your breath with color and other visualizations. The bulk of the meditations focus on the areas, systems, and organs of the body that each chakra governs. By regularly practicing these meditations, you'll get to know each chakra intimately, and you'll create your desired healing effect.

I'll be asking a lot of you in these meditations, especially if you're practicing chakra healing for the first time. But don't worry—I'll provide tips. I'll also explain how to expand the shorter meditations.

CLOSING REFLECTION

Engaging in reflection will help you get comfortable with building your awareness so you can be more in tune with your body and your mind.

After your meditation has concluded, spend about five minutes putting ideas or thoughts that you need to process onto paper. You could also sit with the newly created space of awareness that comes up during meditation. Either way is fine.

Although you won't be cued to spend time in reflection after every meditation, it's a good idea to set two timers: one for the length of the meditation and one for five minutes longer, to give yourself a little buffer before coming back to the real world.

Monkey Mind

The mind can be a land mine of distractions and activity. Your thoughts can race around—much like monkeys swinging from tree to tree. The trees in this case are your emotions and thoughts that are attempting to gain your attention. Originally a Buddhist term meaning "unsettled," "restless," or "indecisive," monkey mind can refer to any mind chatter.

Meditation is not about stopping the chatter—rather, it's about making a choice. Each time you drop into meditation, you have a choice: Allow distractions to pull you out of your space or show up for yourself and go deeper into that space. Instead of jumping from branch to branch, giving anything and everything your attention, make the choice to be present and quiet the chaos.

That choice doesn't mean that you should ignore the chatter. In fact, acknowledging your thoughts can neutralize them, particularly when they include self-doubt.

Giving your mind a task is a good way to transcend thought patterns and processes. One simple technique is to focus on your breath moving in and out of your body. If you become overwhelmed by monkey mind, try incorporating a mantra into your meditation.

Over time, you'll become better at being in the moment. With practice, your thoughts will become less disruptive. Consistency is key here. It's all about training your monkey mind so you can swing gracefully through the trees with patience, compassion, and control.

Before You Begin

Before jumping into your healing practice, there are a few steps that need to be covered. Some of these may seem a bit obvious, but I wouldn't be doing my due diligence as a healer if I didn't include them.

Clearing some time for your meditation is imperative to ensure that your practice is successful. Try setting a daily reminder on your phone to help you establish a meditation habit. Make sure you are comfortable. Eliminate distractions and plan time for reflection before your meditation starts. I'll go over these steps in more detail below.

Do a general check-in with yourself to connect with your current emotions. Make note of any issues so you can develop a loving attitude of self-acceptance each time you practice meditation. And don't worry about whether you're doing it wrong, because there is no wrong way to meditate—I promise!

WHAT YOU'LL NEED

Although meditation doesn't cost money, it does take commitment. The amount of time and effort you put into your practice determines its success.

Outside distractions are all part of the meditation. However, minimize interruptions as much as possible. Make sure you won't be disrupted by any electronics during your sit time. Silence your phone before you begin.

You'll want to keep this book nearby so you can take quick peeks if you get lost during a sit, especially when you're first starting your meditation practice. If you keep a meditation journal, have it easily accessible post-sit.

REFLECTION

It's natural for feelings to come up during meditation. You may need time post-sit to process and integrate these feelings. Creating space for reflection after each meditation is a good practice. I won't give reflection reminders at the end of each meditation, but you'll want to note how you feel.

If some action items have made themselves apparent during your meditation, you can create a to-do list. Drawing or sketching a solution in a journal is another option. A meditation journal can help you succinctly acknowledge whatever came up for you. Plus, it's a great tool for tracking your progress.

On the other hand, it's okay if you feel that not much transpired. It may take a few days or weeks to fully integrate what actually went on behind the scenes during a sit. The solution may be a longer sit.

Reconciling Emotions

When you finish a meditation, you may experience unsettling emotions. When you tap into your subconscious mind, energy begins to move and clear, and you may come away with feelings of frustration, sadness, pain, or anger. Consider meditation an opportunity to integrate and release these feelings.

Although most of us do not like to admit it, pain and discomfort are vital aspects of the human experience. Pain is a response to something occurring in your reality, whereas suffering is the choice to prolong that pain. Both are unpleasant experiences, but they offer a tremendous opportunity for growth, and they remind us of the balance we need to reach our highest potential.

To escape suffering, remember that you have the power to view things from a different perspective. Consistent meditation can help you make that shift. We may not understand why something is happening, but we can do our best to trust, surrender, and accept our emotions—even if they come in the form of pain and suffering.

Taking notes and acknowledging how you feel will help make sense of your healing journey. Consistent reflection will help you build trust in yourself so you'll feel confident listening to your body and mind when they speak—even if they whisper.

Getting Comfortable

You will want to dress in comfortable clothing. Nothing is worse than being pulled away from your meditation by an itchy sweater or too-tight jeans. If you are meditating before work or during lunch, make adjustments that will help you relax, like removing your belt or settling into a cozy chair.

It's not necessary to use a professional meditation cushion, but you will want some back support for comfort. Worrying about discomfort draws attention away from your awareness, so eliminating that issue beforehand will only help facilitate your journey.

When you sit, whether on the floor or in a chair, a straight spine is ideal. If seated on the floor, your legs can be in the lotus position, folded, or straight out in front of you. If you are seated in a chair, your feet should be flat on the floor. I do not recommend crossing your legs or arms because it impedes the flow of energy through your body. If you want to lie down for the meditation, make sure you do so at a time of day when you're likely to remain alert.

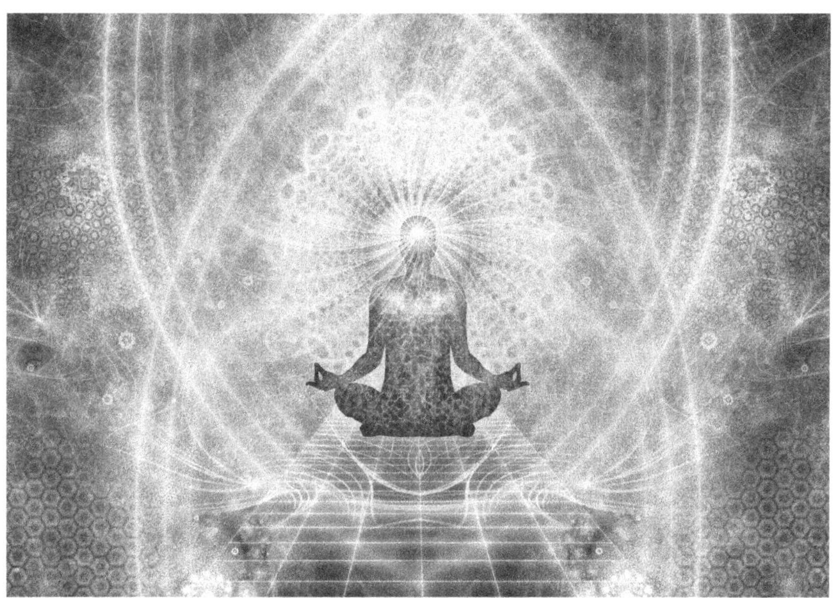

Chapter 3.
Healing Your Chakras

Using the methods of chakra healing, you can treat numerous physical ailments that weren't caused by medical problems or injuries. Pain and diseases that root in mental causes, instead of medical, are called psychosomatic. They are called this because they signal mental distress. They are a sign that your body is overrun by stress hormones and fear hormones. However, it's not enough for you to acknowledge that some of your ailments come from your mind. To understand which particular aspects of your emotional life are struck with blockage and denial and to learn how to release them, you can look into each individual symptom and tie it to the corresponding mental problems.

With this information, you'll understand your body better, and you'll know which of your symptoms result from emotional and spiritual problems.

Headache

If you're suffering from chronic headaches without obvious medical causes, it could be due to the imbalance in your third eye chakra and the crown chakra.

Chronic headaches, followed by sinus pressure, and the pressure in the back part of your head and your eyes, that spread across your forehead, are the most typical sign of the disharmony in the third eye chakra.

These pains are a signal that you are mainly focusing on the intellectual and neglecting the spiritual aspects of your existence. You may be afraid of your spiritual aspects. Because of this, you are ignoring your intuitive hints and abandoning the wisdom of your third eye.

Many times, your instincts tell you to do things that seem to go against logic. You feel these signals, but you are afraid that acting on them would be risky.

For example, if you unconsciously feel like you should quit your job, but there is no new job in sight, you might be ignoring this instinct.

Subconsciously, your third eye knows the things that are beyond your conscious knowledge. It might be signaling to you that the better opportunity is coming your way. Or, you may be in the presence of a person you unconsciously know has a negative effect on you. But, you are ignoring the intuitive signals to stay away from that person.

On the other hand, a headache at the top center of your head is often a sign of the imbalance in the crown chakra. This type of headache suggests difficulty trusting the intuitive signs regarding your life path.

You may fear that acting and living in accordance with the Divine signals will lead to something risky or irresponsible. This results from having difficulties in seeing a larger picture and cultivating your faith in yourself and in the Divine.

Fatigue

Fatigue is detrimental to your energy focus and concentration which all results in low motivation. If you are someone who usually overwork themselves into exhaustion, you are overloading your solar plexus chakra and your power center is being overstimulated.

If you're suffering from fatigue, it is most likely due to the imbalance in the crown chakra and the solar plexus chakra. The ongoing exhaustion that only increases and doesn't go away after rest, with a constant feeling of weariness and low energy, signals chakra imbalance.

This can happen if you are associating achievement and self-esteem with the quality of your performance. If you feel like failing to deliver quality performance makes you unworthy, it can have a negative effect on your solar plexus chakra. This is often followed by low self-esteem, depression, and loss of faith in the Divine.

Stomach disorders

Pain and uncomfortable symptoms in your stomach come from the imbalance of the solar plexus chakra. Diseases related to stomach include diarrhea, constipation, intestinal problems, ulcers, acid reflux, and many others. If you are certain that you haven't eaten any foods that might have upset your stomach, or that there haven't been any physical injuries that might have caused these symptoms, you can inspect your solar plexus chakra to see if it's out of balance.

Pain in your stomach can often result from the feeling of powerlessness, a sense of overwhelm, a perception that you are losing control of your life, feeling intimidated or having low self-respect. If you went through significant changes in your life, like a divorce, problematic relationships with other people, or a loss of a job, these experiences could have produced a lot of anger, resentment, guilt, and other toxic emotions.

If your self-esteem is compromised, you will have a very toxic combination of negative feelings towards other people and yourself. The key to resolving this is to forgive both yourself and others, as well as admitting that there is no reason to place blame on anyone.

To overcome stomach pains related to the solar plexus chakra, you can apply the solar plexus meditation or use essential oils to treat your stomach area with more kindness and compassion.

Psychosomatic digestive problems arise from your problems with processing stress. They are a sign that you are ignoring to resolve problems in your daily life. When you're not processing daily stresses, they become suppressed. You are resorting to emotional avoidance.

As a result of this, you are closing your solar plexus chakra because you don't want to deal with problems.

This is dangerous because your solar plexus is the center of your personal power. When you avoid confronting problems, you are shutting yourself out from using your personal power to solve them. As a result of this, you feel frightened, powerless, and your self-esteem is low. The only solution for this is addressing the things that are bothering you.

Detachment

When you feel disconnected and detached from yourself and the world around you that means that you've closed your heart chakra. In this state, you abandon your passions and you give up everything that makes you happy and fulfilled.

The first sign of the imbalance of the heart chakra is the lack of connection with others. You may feel the need to be alone, which can turn into isolation. When you feel the need to isolate from others, it means that you are shutting yourself out.

You want to feel happy and joyful, but it seems like you are no longer able to. You are out of touch with everything that makes you happy. This can lead to depression.

You may even be disconnected from your physical body and unable to feel the physical sensations before they become overwhelming. For example, you don't notice symptoms of illnesses before they become too intense. You start living on autopilot, disengaging from your true self.

Detachment is best treated with mindfulness. Start looking into everything that makes you happy. Focus on gratefulness and put more effort into spending time with your friends and family. First, you need to establish a good connection with yourself, which can be done through meditation and other self-care practices.

Depression

While physical trauma can induce depression, it is mainly a mental state in which a person's negative beliefs prevail over the positive perceptions of oneself and life. What gives people a sense of purpose, meaning, and a feeling that they belong in the world is faith in God. Having faith in God is essential because none of us are truly in control over anything, including our own lives and our own bodies.

What keeps us going is the faith that there is general positivity in the world and that things will work out for us. We rely on this faith even when outside manifestation speaks otherwise.

Due to traumatic events, a problematic childhood, or a combination of multiple factors, negative beliefs can prevail over positive thoughts. When you have experiences like these, your heart chakra and your crown chakra will fall out of balance.

Your heart chakra is in charge of being open to love. It is in charge of feeling worthy of love and wanting to love others selflessly and unconditionally. Related to that is the crown chakra, which embodies your relationship with the Divine. That relationship is primarily a relationship of love. It requires faith.

When you fall into depression, you essentially lose faith in love. Not only in love, you lose faith in "good," which resonates with losing faith in God. This is an unconscious process that might not manifest in conscious thoughts due to blockage. You don't want to admit that you've lost your faith and you block out these feelings.

As a result, you feel hopeless and undeserving of anything good. In this state, both your crown and heart chakra will close or constrict. You will experience continuous sadness, feeling hopeless, and empty. You will have trouble finding pleasure and feel like your life is not worth living.

This condition also affects your appetite and sleep, which puts you in an even worse situation. Your energy comes from the foods you consume, and when you're neglecting your diet, you are also depriving yourself of the source of your life energy. You become energetically depleted.

The crown chakra, when out of balance, produces a feeling of loneliness. In extreme situations, this can lead to suicidal thoughts, and eventually suicide.

When you are feeling depressed, focus on working on balancing your heart chakra first. Your heart chakra helps you open up to love. It helps you open up to the sense of safety. It also helps you accept the idea that you are worthy of unconditional love and that there's nothing that you have to do to deserve it.

Your crown chakra, which should only be treated when the root chakra is in good shape, is now in need of love. To work on your crown chakra, devote to religious, mindful, or spiritual practices. You should work on your relationship with the Divine, in whichever ways you practice spiritual beliefs.

Make sure to address any unconscious anger towards God. Most people find it hard to grasp that while God is a cosmic force that teaches you about right and wrong, He is also endlessly forgiving. When people feel guilty, they also feel like God thinks they are guilty, and God is judging them. This is never true. The Divine force is the force of unconditional forgiveness.

If you feel angry with God, you actually feel angry at yourself. You assume that God is angry at you because you didn't act according to his/her/its teachings.

In this case, you should contemplate on God's imminent and unconditional love for every person. You can do this by reading scriptures or talking to a religious teacher who will explain how the Divine looks at people, and why it always forgives.

Grief

Loss can cause constriction and the closing of the heart chakra.

Grief is a feeling that results from losing something that is precious to us. With relationships, jobs, and material goods, it's easier to cope with grief because there is a lesser significance to the loss. However, some losses, like the death of loved ones and children are very hard to cope with. There's no replacement for what we're missing, and relief seems impossible to find.

Loss can very easily block your heart chakra, causing you to grief for a long time. This causes the feeling of loneliness, hopelessness, and the cultivation of bitterness.

Grief is commonly followed by isolation. In some cases, isolation is a good idea for you to rejuvenate and pick yourself up. However, if isolation results from the unwillingness to reconnect with the world, it can become harmful.

Your heart chakra connects you to the sense of self-love and love for others. Grief can cause you to lose faith in love, and even choose to detach from it, to avoid feeling pain. The cure for grief is reconnecting with your own inner feeling of self-love, love for others, and the outside world. If you feel like grief has become toxic for you, there are many healthy ways for you to reconnect.

You can start by practicing self-love and self-care and then move to connect with people, plants, and animals. If a heartbreak makes it hard for you to reconnect with your loved ones, you can start by connecting with plants and animals. Gradually, this connection will help you open up to connecting with people.

Guilt

An overwhelming feeling of guilt may constrict your solar plexus and the sacral plexus chakra. When you feel profoundly guilty of having done something wrong, whether or not this perception is true, you detach yourself from feeling pleasure. You deny yourself pleasure because you feel undeserving of it.

This can cause you to repress your sexuality, emotions, and overall detach from doing things that make you happy. Guilt results in the loss of will to express yourself in healthy ways.

To heal guilt, practice meditations for solar and sacral plexus chakras, and also work on healthy self-expression. Healing from guilt means being able to assume the responsibility for your actions but releasing the feeling of inadequacy.

No one benefits from you feeling guilty. The guilt itself doesn't repair any harm that you may have done. You can work towards amending whatever harm you have done if there's room for it. If not, you can only work to learn from your mistakes. However, making a mistake doesn't mean that you no longer deserve to be happy.

Anxiety

Anxiety affects all chakras depending on the type of strain you're exposed to. Everyday life often entails a moderate amount of anxiety. However, long-term anxiety followed by constant stress can have a negative impact on your health. You will become more vulnerable to triggers. Within minutes of a triggering situation, you can find yourself in a state of panic.

Most often, anxiety affects your crown and heart chakra. This happens when you start to feel like God doesn't have your back. The third eye chakra causes anxiety due to fear of the unknown, and distrust of your intuition.

This can severely impact your quality of life. When your throat chakra is out of harmony, you will be anxious about expressing your opinions and holding your truth. As a result, everything you have to say and the things that burdens you will be repressed.

Holding on to past hurts can block your heart chakra and cause anxiousness because you feel disconnected from your own feelings. Intimidation and overwhelming fear, be it in the area of work, finance, or relationships, with the added pressure to perform perfectly, causes your solar plexus chakra to fall out of balance.

With sacral plexus chakra, anxiety results from feeling guilty and ashamed to confess your needs and insecurities. Over time, these built-up tensions can have a profoundly debilitating impact on your life. Anxiety also touches your root chakra in the form of feeling insecure and unsafe.

To heal anxiety using chakra healing, you should examine your insecurities in all aspects of your inner being, starting from the bottom to the top.

Screen all of your chakras and determine which areas are a source of negative energy. Then, start by practicing grounding to insure yourself that the Earth is supporting you. Proceed to heal your chakras using meditation, crystals, and essential oils. Focus on releasing your fears in regard to all issues that are relevant to the chakras.

Anger

Anger mostly affects your root chakra, but it also touches on the other energy centers as well. Anger, in its core, is a healthy feeling that drives you to stand up for yourself, establish boundaries, act, and initiate change.

However, anger can also become a tool for you to repress sadness. When this happens, you are using anger to defend yourself from the inner feeling of sadness and hopelessness. Fear can also be the root of anger and your using anger away to the fence yourself being afraid. While anger resonates deeply with the root chakra, it affects all other chakras. If you are angry at God for the suffering of bad faith, this touches on your crown chakra.

Your third eye also becomes affected because due to this, you lose faith in your own intuition. You're out of touch with an inner sense of emotional intelligence. You will become unable to trust yourself, and as a result, you no longer trust the world and the Divine. You also start to distrust your community and your loved ones. The key to healing anger is to inspect the underlying feelings.

For example, if you are angry for not standing up for yourself, the solution might be in balancing your solar plexus chakra. However, if you feel anger, to defend yourself from fear and sadness, the solutions are to treat your heart chakra and your sacral chakra. These chakras open you up to forgiveness and love.

If your anger roots in feeling burdened, then it's possible that you are holding in some truths that need to be said. These truths can relate to many areas of your life, from unpleasant things that you need to admit to yourself to deeply hidden truths you want to reveal to the world. If guilt and shame stop you from doing this, you need to learn how to overcome them. Only when you start going through life fully authentic to your inner truth will you be able to relieve the anger and live in peace.

Chapter 4.
The Third Eye And
Your Psychic Awakening

The third eye is the main ascension space when you are preparing to reach enlightenment. You cannot begin to even wonder what it means to be enlightened if your third eye is blocked, congested, or stagnant. The third eye is the seat of perception, intuition, and "clear knowing," and it is how we are wonderfully able to connect to our dreams and visions in a more profound way.

You can live your whole life without ever knowing the quality of what it feels like to be connected to this part of yourself, and many people describe it as feeling high without having any drugs or alcohol. It can be the way that you ask yourself to pursue a higher mind so that you can live a fuller life, which sometimes means letting go of the status quo and not trying so hard to "fit in."

Answering the call of the third eye isn't as hard as people might suggest, and when you are open to it and have created awareness about it, you can begin to use simple tools to help yourself realize the power of the third eye in your overall chakra healing experience.

Mental Relaxation Tools to Awaken Higher Consciousness

Your mind is a machine, constantly computing and deciding, deciphering and learning, and even feeling skeptical or judgmental. Your third eye doesn't have time for all of that and will have a harder time being open if you are closed off to it with your mental thoughts. The third eye is energy, and it is the beginning of your worlds becoming one, between the physical and the spiritual.

The mental attitudes and beliefs that people adopt in early life, or adapt to within their culture or community, can be very limiting to the third eye and so as you prepare to work with opening this energy, it is important to find ways to relax your mind in order to awaken higher consciousness.

Mindfulness is a form of meditation that can be performed in any situation. It is an act of being totally conscious of everything that you are experiencing at the moment without letting your mind wander too far into the past or the future. It keeps your mind free of anxious or worrisome thoughts because you are working only to engage with the experience you are having right now.

Mindfulness can take some practice, and it is incredibly simple to learn. All you have to do is follow these simple guidelines:

- Focus and concentrate on what you are working with right now.

- Don't get caught up in making assumptions or having too many opinions about the experience. Try to just enjoy a quiet mind while you take in the situation or surroundings.

- Find the openings you see in your intuition and let them guide you forward. Trust your instinct.

- When your mind starts to churn too much, or worry what others might be doing, thinking and feeling, return yourself to what you are doing and give it added focus.

- Breathe, inhales and exhales, steadily and calmly.

- Give yourself over to going with the flow and don't try to control the situation or the outcomes.

- Visualize your inner world as it is making contact with your outer world and see how the two can be together. Practice seeing more than what your eyes can see naturally.

These simple guidelines are just some of the basics of practicing mindfulness. When you are working to incorporate a higher consciousness level of thinking and processing information, you have to be able to let go of control and just bear witness to reality. It will show you what you need to know, rather than imposing an opinion, belief, or attitude upon it.

This is the platform for thinking from a higher state of being, and it will naturally occur that your third eye will expand and become more alive to your overall thought process naturally as a result of this attitude or process.

The Art of Creative Visualization

To be able to see with your eyes closed is the gift of the third eye. It is not something reserved only for the enlightened. It is possible for any person, no matter what level of awakening they are involved with at the moment. All it takes is a little effort and a few minutes of your time to practice this useful skill.

Creative visualization feels a lot like what it is like to dream. When you go to sleep at night, and you can recall your dreams, there are usually moving pictures, images, sensations, and even thoughts or words. When you are creatively visualizing something out of the dream state, you are activating your higher mind and deeper consciousness.

There are plenty of people who already know how to do this and have always known how to close their eyes and imagine a far off and fantastical landscape full of whatever comes to mind. With a little practice, it can become even more detailed and elaborate, and you will find a greater opening with your capabilities with your psychic visions and ability to see beyond what is visible to the naked eye.

It is this skill that will help you see your chakras more clearly and be more open to understanding the visions that come up or resurface from past experiences so that you know what you need to let go of clearly. The path of awakening the third eye can be advanced when you practice this technique. Here are the simple guidelines to follow when you are practicing creative visualization:

- Be open to anything that might surface without judgment or criticism.

- Let go of thought patterns and cycles that you might easily get stuck in (ex: "I can't," "that isn't real/possible," "It doesn't even make any sense," etc.).

- Teach yourself your own methods and avoid looking online or in books for a guide to help you connect with your third eye. The point is that you are connecting to your own unique intuition and identity.

- Visualize things simple at first and then more elaborately as you get better at seeing the minute details.

- Practice traveling to other "inner landscapes" and worlds to help show yourself the metaphorical and symbolic path that you need to travel.

- Design your worlds to be places that you can return to over and over again to help yourself along your healing path.

- Use your thoughts and feelings to direct the course of your creative visualization. It will help you to better identify what chakras will need the most healing, balance, or strengthening.

These simple guidelines are just to give you a platform to begin your own creative work. The journey of awakening the third eye is unique to the individual and will be different for everyone. It is important not to get too boxed into other people's views or perspectives about the "right" or "wrong" way to open your third eye (or any other chakras, for that matter).

Creative visualization is a portal to help you understand your own inner truth as well as to finding your path to universal consciousness and enlightenment.

Power of Psychic Awareness Through the Third Eye

There are no limits to what the human mind is capable of. We are only limited by our beliefs and ideas about what it all is supposed to be or look like. Awakening, the third eye asks you to let go of all of your preconceived notions of reality and to step into a new way of seeing all life on the planet.

The power of psychic awareness will make it challenging for you to know anything the way that you knew it before. It causes a great shift in your ability to "see" and "know" the truth about all areas of your life, which will, in turn, cause a lot of change, even when it is uncomfortable. You may not know it yet, but when you begin to ascend into your psychic knowledge, you will look at your world with a new set of eyes, and it will suddenly feel like everything you are doing in your life right now is "off" and needs to change or be resolved.

This great transformation happens very quickly, and many people will even avoid the cost of letting it unfold naturally out of fear of such a big life change or shift in consciousness and identity. There are certainly ways that you can help this experience unfold in a healthier and more comfortable way and here are just a few tips to help you understand that process:

- Give up anything that no longer makes you feel like yourself.

- Look for ways to explore your psychic awareness by listening to your inner codes and messages that come up. It is your intuition and inner knowing speaking to you. Keep a journal or a record of these psychic thoughts.

- Bring yourself into a state of trance or meditation on a daily or regular basis to help you expand your consciousness more effectively.

- Take a moment to listen to your gut reactions and instincts before you make a choice or speak any words to someone or yourself.

- Denial is not a helpful tool, and so if you ask these questions and receive a response, do not deny it, no matter how far-fetched it may seem.

- Collaborate with other methods of psychic practice, such as divination, scrying, tarot card reading, crystal empowerment of the third eye, etc.

- Release any beliefs that suggest that being psychic isn't real or true.

The moment you begin to embrace your ability to just "know" you are giving yourself the opening to awakening your psychic abilities more than ever before. What are those psychic abilities? They manifest differently for everyone, but here is a list of some possibilities:

- Prophetic dreams and prophecies

- The ability to see what is about to happen as it is about to happen

- Welcoming the presence of spirit guides and other "ethereal helpers."

- Clairvoyance and clairsentience

- Being able to predict possible outcomes in a detailed way

- Journeying in mind to other dimensions of reality, or astral travel

- Being able to speak to energies on the "other side."

- Reading auras and being able to see the light and coloration of the auras

- Being able to read another person's energy and interpret what they are not saying out loud

- Telepathy

- And more!

Psychic awareness takes a lot of personal growth, stamina, and ability to see beyond the third dimension of reality. It can take you years to uncover the depths of your psychic powers and path, and if you put in the work to truly know yourself in this way, then you can advance your soulful awakening even faster than if you just did a few things here and a couple of things there.

Understanding Enlightenment

Enlightenment simply means that you are awakening to your whole light source and power as a person. It is a connection to the universally divine energies inherent in all things and all nature. You don't have to be a yoga guru or someone who lives and breathes the philosophies of Eastern religions in order to know enlightenment. It is a different path for every person with different ways of traveling throughout life.

There are a lot of ways that people will feel confused about what enlightenment is because they are looking for perfection. It is not a state of perfection that equals enlightenment, but rather a state of truth within your own being. If you are resistant to your own truth, then you are not likely to become fully enlightened, and in order to get to that connection with yourself, you have to let go of what you think and believe that the world wants you to be. You can live your whole life exhausting your true purpose by trying to fit in the way other people do or try to.

Enlightenment is a growth experience, and it will never fit into a list of rules or a checklist. It is an ongoing process that delivers you to your highest and purest form of consciousness and even that required continuous fine-tuning and exploration. There really is no endpoint to the journey of self-discovery, and it will only limit you if you think, feel or believe that if only you could just make it that point, everything will be great forever.

It simply won't work that way, and having an awakened mind means that you are already in awareness of that simple truth and reality. Your third eye and your psychic ascension is the path that opens you to becoming enlightened and working forward toward living your life by your inner light and source energy. And that is really what healing the chakras and awakening is all about in the first place.

Chapter 5.
The Ways To Protect Yourself During Third Eye Activation

The third eye activation is a powerful process. It makes you more receptive. You will attract energies around you. However, you cannot have real control over the kind of energies with which you may come in contact. You simply become the receiver of energies. This can pose a problem.

The positive energies will bring peace and tranquility. They will make you strong and blissful. However, negative energies can have a stronger but negative impact. To this end, it is important that you protect yourself. You must become aware of the energies around you. You must choose the place of practice carefully. You should also work to seal your aura for getting better protection against negative energies.

Neglecting these important aspects can have serious consequences on your physical, mental, as well as spiritual health. Enabling psychic protection against negative energies is the best way to avoid these issues.

The places of meditation, the lifestyle you follow, and even the kind of clothes you wear have important roles to play in your protection. Proper attention to all these aspects will help you in ensuring proper protection. We will now discuss the main things that you need to take into consideration.

The Place

The place of meditation has a very important role to play in ensuring your protection. We are surrounded by all kinds of energies. There are positive energies that help us in our endeavors. There are negative energies that push us down or corner us. The whole concept of things and places being lucky or unlucky isn't just a misconception. When positive energies in a place are dominant, that place becomes lucky. It helps you in becoming successful. You become more energetic and alive. Your entrepreneurial skills get sharp. Your risk-taking abilities become stronger. Your ability to judge people, things, and circumstances gets better. You feel rejuvenated and healthy. However, if the place is dominated by negative energies, things are exactly the opposite.

Therefore, ignoring the significance of the place is not a very prudent thing. We are not the first to roam on this earth. Several people have walked, lived, and died in the same place where we live at present. A part of their energy is left behind. Accumulation of such energies has a profound effect on the nature of that place.

This earth is the place from which we all have originated. It is also a very powerful source of energy. It is full of energies that are so powerful that your body can never react to them positively. Such energies keep leaking from the fault lines. If you are at a place which is contaminated by such energies, then they will have a negative impact on you. Fear, health, and psychological problems are only some type of issues that can be faced.

In the past, people gave great significance to the earth's energies. They had the luxury to move things around. Space was ample. They could shift even a home if it rested on such fault lines. Modern lifestyle doesn't permit you this luxury. Living spaces have become smaller. Homes have become so expensive that shifting them in search of a feasible option isn't an option anymore. However, there are other remedies like Feng Shui, Vastu Shashtra, dowsing, house healing, and other such practices that can help you in cultivating positive energies. You will be able to identify the places in your home filled with negative energies. Such places can be easily avoided, and you can do constructive practices elsewhere. Like fields of negative energies, homes also have energy wells. These are the areas of positive energy. You can identify these areas and utilize them to your advantage.

Earth ray lines have been known to be a reason for several health issues. Our ancestor's associated cot deaths with such ray lines. People sleeping on these ray lines are known to be prone to joint problems, heart conditions, migraine headaches, and other such ailments. Frequent and unexplained bed-wetting is also attributed to these ray lines. If you are constantly having bad dreams while sleeping in the same place, then changing the direction or position of your bed can help. Insomnia or difficulty in sleeping can be due to this problem.

Such energies also impact your meditation and its results. While you are in a meditative state, your aura expands, and it starts communicating with the energies around it. Excessive influence of negative energies can lead to fear and visualization of negative imagery. It can leave you in a fearful state and make longer meditations difficult. That's why it is important to find a place that is more conducive.

Once you start meditation, your sense of perception will become sharper. You will be able to feel such energies strongly. If you feel that meditating at any particular place is getting difficult, you must change the place. You can also take the help of professional dowsers, house healers, or Feng Shui to balance the energies.

Work on Yourself

A healthy body and a balanced mind are the best defense

Attacking the weak is the best strategy and we all know this. Negativity will engulf the weak of mind and body first. So, you must always focus on having a healthy body and a balanced mind. If you remain healthy and sane, negative forces will not be able to influence you easily. You must adopt a healthy lifestyle to remain protected.

A balanced lifestyle and mindset are the first requisite for any such practice. If you are stepping into your practice with a negative outlook, the results won't be very promising. Your journey would remain bumpy, and you would face several impediments on the way.

A healthy body is a strong foundation for success. You will be able to face your fears with strength and overpower the roadblocks easily. The protection techniques will work in any condition, but a healthy lifestyle will help you in many ways.

Third eye activation is a spiritual journey, but it has to be carried out through your physical body; and therefore, you can never ignore the importance of your physicality. You must take steps to ensure that you remain healthy and focused. Following a healthy lifestyle will take you a long way in this process.

Sleep and rest are important

An exhausted body is weak and prone to the influence of negative energies. If you are taxing yourself too much or not getting enough sleep, then you will become empty. This state will be easier to overpower. Some people start meditation and want to achieve things very quickly. They undermine this important concept and face dire consequences.

You must ensure that you are getting ample time to rest and have proper sleep. Lack of rest and sleep will make you weak. Your energy field will also get weak, and your protection cover will fade away.

Meditation is the art of relaxation. However, it is not a substitute for rest and sleep. You must give yourself an ample amount of time to remain fresh and rejuvenated. If you are facing a time crunch, then you should adjust your meditation time accordingly. It is not only the time of meditation practice that matters but your consistency, too.

You can practice at short intervals. Take some time out in the morning when you wake up. This is the best time to practice as your body is relaxed and your mind is fresh. It will also give a great kickstart to your day. In the evening, when you return from work, you can devote some time to meditation. This will help you in relaxing, and you will also sleep better.

Do not try to rush the process by overtaxing yourself in the beginning. It is a way of life that you will have to manage on a long-term basis. Finding a sustainable way to do it is always the best strategy.

Focusing on this simple aspect will help you in remaining steadfast, and it will also prevent you from the influence of negative energies.

A balanced diet

A simple fact of life is that we become what we eat. The food that we eat has a very strong influence on our lives. If you are eating an unbalanced diet, it will have a negative influence on your physical and mental wellbeing, as well as your spiritual consciousness. The activation of the third eye also gets heavily influenced by the kind of diet you have.

This is among the key reasons that the monks have very simple, yet healthy meals. They focus on supplying a healthy mix of macronutrients to their body. They eat the foods that can be easily processed by the body.

In this modern way of life where processed food has taken over the natural diet, it would be unwise to prescribe any strict eating regimen. However, you should stay away from an unbalanced diet. You must always eat the right mix of macronutrients that supply you with needed energy. Following diet plans or strict calorie control will expose you to negative energies as you become weak. It is a very unwise thing to do. You can also get the same results by having a diet that supplies all the required nutrients and eliminates the junk food that leads to excess weight. Whatever the diet plan you follow, you must ensure that it is nutritious.

Some people also get misled by the notion that fasting help in meditation. There is no doubt that fasting has a profound impact on meditation. It helps you in becoming calmer as the food always keeps reacting to your body and generates several kinds of reactions. However, fasting is only beneficial when it is done in a controlled manner. You cannot simply start fasting all of a sudden and expect positive results. In fact, the whole process would become counterproductive. Your mind will remain busy with the thoughts of food.

Fasting should only be done as a part of detoxification. It helps in cleaning your body of the toxic stuff and should not be over-stretched. Creating irregular gaps in your meal will only harm your efforts. Regular meals have a great role in reinforcing your astral body. You feel more content and vital.

You must focus on foods that have a lot of antioxidants and help in fighting free radicals. Eating easily digestible food is always the best way to remain healthy and fit. Complex foods, especially red meat, take a lot of time to digest. It also promotes the growth of negative energies in your body. You should try to avoid it as much as possible.

Remain joyful

Sorrow or grief are dark emotions. They attract negative energies a lot. Somewhere deep down there is a grudge building up. The development of positive energies becomes difficult in such a state. Happiness, laughter, and positivity, on the other hand, keep the dark energies at bay. You become strong and remain protected.

You must cultivate happiness. Try to remain cheerful. If you are unhappy about a few things in the past, try to forgive and forget them. Moving on will be easier for you. Moving on the path of third eye awakening with baggage from the past is not a healthy thing. Joy and peace are important in life. In fact, happiness has been the ultimate goal of the majority of people who have walked on this earth. Sadness and depression only weigh you down. Make your choice prudently.

Don't intoxicate yourself

The intoxication of any kind may give you a temporary relief from the problems of this world, but it cannot be a permanent solution. In fact, it isn't a solution at all. Problems generally become bigger when you come out of a hangover. You must stay away from avoid this scenario.

Drugs and alcohol have become quite popular. They cause hallucinations and make you see an imaginary world which you may like. However, they take you far away from reality.

Drugs and alcohol can be dangerous while you are on the path of third eye activation. You may hallucinate and have false visualizations. They also make you weak and incapable of exercising any control. You become weak and may become influenced by negative energies. You must stay away from them to remain protected.

Some Effective Ways to Manage Energies

Choose your colors wisely

The color you wear will have a profound impact on the amount of energy you absorb. Light colors do not absorb energy. This will help you a lot in staying safe from the influence of negative energies. This is one of the reasons white color is the preferred color for meditation. It reflects negative energies.

Dark colors attract and absorb energy. If you are wearing dark colors while doing your meditation, then the chances of coming in contact with the dark energies increase.

Find a positive place for meditation

The place of meditation has a very strong impact. A place with an excess of negative energies will always give you a hard time in meditation. You will be able to feel an intense pressure. There will be distractions and you will find it difficult to concentrate for long. If you find yourself in any such situation, then the chances are that you are sitting on a fault line. Shifting the place of meditation even by a few feet can make a lot of difference.

You can take remedial steps for correcting the flow of energy, yet fighting it for long will not yield great results. Shift the place of your meditation and find a corner that has a positive flow of energy or an energy well. Such a place will have a soothing impact and you will be able to meditate effortlessly.

Wash your hands

Once you start meditation, your sense of perception of the outside energy forces increases. You are able to feel their interaction with your body. You will be able to feel the extra pressure on your hands. You will become aware of energy building up around you. These realizations will become common. All this happens because you start attracting more energy toward yourself.

Whenever you feel any such pressure in your hands, you must wash them thoroughly under running water. It will increase your perception. It will also keep you safe from such energies.

Purify the room

The presence of negative and positive energies is beyond your control in any place. However, managing as best as you can is always in your interest. If you feel that your home or the place of meditation has a high concentration of negative energies, then you can take some proactive steps to balance these energies.

Burn incense or candles

Burning incense or candles have a positive impact on the energies. You can make the positive energies stronger by this method. It also helps in purifying the room. It gets filled with positivity and smells great. You will be able to meditate for longer.

Hot and cold treatment

Creating a temperature variation in the room is also a way to deal with the flow of energy. You can use heaters to make your room as warm as possible, and let it become cold afterward. Creating a temperature difference in the room helps immensely.

Get in sync with the lunar cycle

The moon has a deep impact on the energies on the earth. It generates a great force. Even the oceans and currents do not remain unaffected by the influence of the moon. The behavior of energies varies on the full moon and new moon. You must consider this factor.

A full moon night is the best time to meditate. You will feel an explosion of energy during this period. It is a very suitable time for intellectual realization. The chances of third eye awakening are very high in this phase of the month. You must make the best use of this time.

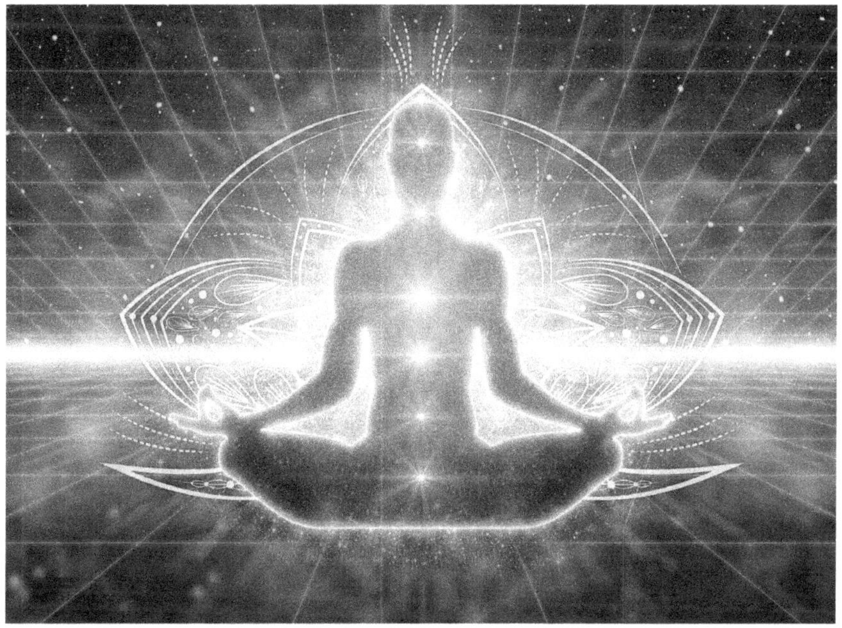

Chapter 6.
The Effect Oy Yoga
On Chakras

Everybody loves good health. More than anything, physical wellness contributes largely to our overall well-being. Therefore it is not surprising that people place a priority on their physical well-being. One of the many ways that people take care of their health is exercise. There are various other ways such as the constant intake of a balanced diet, lot of rest, frequent medical checkups and many more. Many find it easy to discipline themselves, their body and their appetite. This is done basically with the aim of keeping the body fit and healthy. One of these many ways of keeping the body fit is Yoga. Just like exercise or diet, Yoga is a combination of many different activities, and these activities are most effective when they are repeated again and again. The continuity enhances its effects in the body. Beyond exercise, yoga is not only targeted at the body but it is very important to the mind.

If over time, you have practiced yoga, beyond doubt, you have experienced its benefits. It could be evident in your sleep, your health generally or your muscles and bones. It is quite easier to explain these benefits to an ardent believer in yoga, especially one who has practiced it time and over again. These same explanations may add complications to your discussion with someone who has never practiced yoga. Yoga has gone beyond a locally accepted practice and it is beginning to enjoy the attention it deserves from researchers. Scientists have started pinning down evidences on the effects of Yoga on health, how it works to ease pain and aches and most importantly, how it keeps the individual away from frequent hospital visits. These scientific explanations make it easier to draw more people to their mats. The practice of Yoga makes you more flexible, increases the strength of your muscles, perfects your posture, prevents cartilage and joint breakdown, increases your blood flow, increases your heart rate, drops your blood pressure and helps you establish a healthy lifestyle amongst other benefits.

Beyond the benefits of yoga to your body, there are other benefits that are more related to your mind and indeed, your overall well-being. Yoga helps you focus. This practice gives your mind room to relax, builds your inner strength, increases your self-esteem, and brings you into guidance. You would be learning from an expert, a yoga teacher who already has experiences and knows how best to employ yoga to your advantage. It also helps you build self-awareness and improves the quality of your relationships. Yoga helps you understand yourself better, this understanding is then extended to others.

There is no overemphasizing the numerous benefits of yoga, on your body, mind and relationships. You may be yet to determine if it is truly beneficial to all aspects of your body and life. Beyond doubt, it is. Yoga takes care of your body to the least of the details, including the chakras. How amazing is it that there is a single practice that can help you this much? If nothing has convinced you about yoga, let this do the work. Yoga does an amazing job on your chakras.

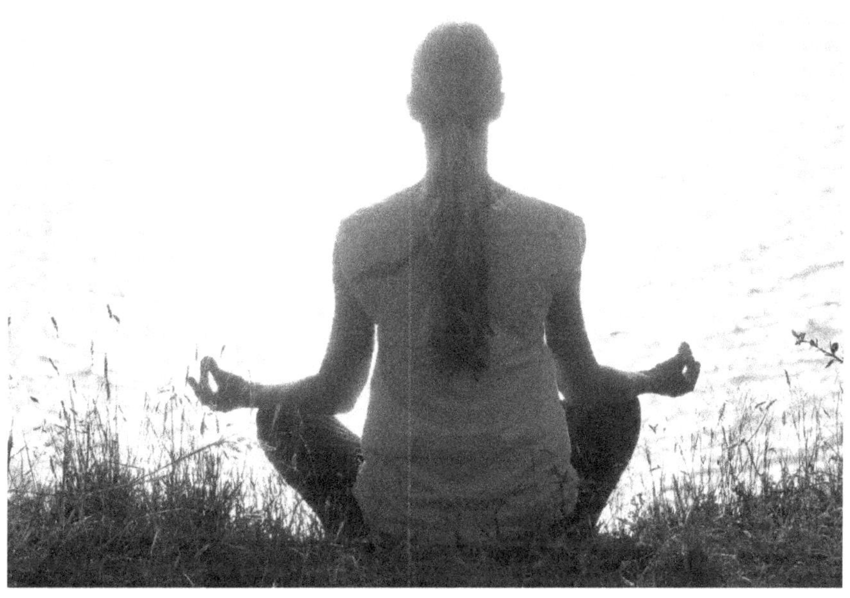

YOGA AND THE CHAKRAS

While you practice yoga, there is a life force energy that goes through the body within a number of channels. The life force energy is the 'prana ', while the series of channels are known as 'nadis. The channels are divided into parts at various points of amplified energy. These are the chakras. Each is responsible for certain responses to stimuli, certain values and behavior in our lives. Some of these life issues directed by the chakras include love and communication. There are other such issues. The chakras are also responsible for regulating different body systems, one of which is the skeletal system. Each chakra has a connection to a particular color along the rainbow, as well as a specific element, mantra.

It is possible for the series of channels to get blocked. When this happens, the chakras also stagnate. At this point, the life force reduces in pace. This can reduce the health of our body, mind and emotions. What yoga does in this event is to purify and re-energize the channels, the chakras. The life force then continues to flow freely. It is a fact that yoga is one of the easiest ways to put each chakra into balance. This is because it creates alignment in the body. As you balance your body through different yoga postures, your body begins to regain stability. This balance causes the chakras to align. This has effects on the sets of behavior you exhibit. It also makes unlearning obsolete habits and values easier. Yoga practices train us to channel our energies correctly, applying pressure where we should and releasing tension where necessary. This practice is particularly important to the chakra because they are responsible for many other issues relating to our total well-being.

Beyond the general effects of stretching and aligning the chakras, yoga improves the functionality of each chakra.

YOGA AND THE ROOT CHAKRA

The root chakra is responsible for your emotional stability. It helps you feel grounded and keeps you assured that you can cope with any situation that comes along your way. Surely, you do not want to go about without this kind of confidence. It is the root chakra that supplies this balance to your body. The serenity and satisfaction that comes from this balance is desirable. It is good for you and the people around you. Yoga helps you find this balance in your root chakra. This chakra is situated at the lowest part of the spine, the pelvic floor and the first three vertebrae. This chakra supplies the feeling of being deeply rooted in our lives.

It is all about finding balance. The root chakra acts as the balance base for the individual's body and life. You are not supposed to retain excess energy in this chakra and you also have to gather enough energy here. Your need to release and gain energy in the Muladhara is taken care of by yoga practices. Yoga helps you retain as much energy as you need in the root chakra. Realizing the fact that excess energy is bad for you, you can also shed the excess through yoga. The balance the yoga helps you achieve sets the ground for true transformation and personal growth in you. Some yoga postures that help you find balance in this region include Sukhasana, Balasana, Malasana, Uttanasana, Mountain pose, Sun salutations, Anjaneyasana, etc.

YOGA AND THE SACRAL CHAKRA

The sacral chakra located at the inner pelvis and lower belly helps the body to achieve flow, flexibility and fun. Here is where your relationship with yourself and other people is coordinated. Yoga opens up your chakra and this opening and alignment allow each chakra to operate at the best frequency. What would you do without the beautiful relationships in your life, what about the way you look into the mirror and you are totally in love with who you see? Do you know the amount of work it takes to understand yourself and the people around you?

You give yourself a better chance at these things as you practice yoga. The level of relaxation that yoga allows in your body and mind opens up this chakra and allows you to convert and harness the energy here to creativity and an amazing amount of understanding, first of yourself and then, other people. You gain a deeper understanding of your default reactions and emotions. Of course, the essence of self-awareness and healthy relationships cannot be over emphasized, as this is highly consequential to our mental health. When the sacral chakra is not aligned with others, some physical conditions can be visible. They include low back pain, urinary tract infections, impotence, ovarian cysts and some other reproductive issue.

Poses like Dvipada Pitham (bridge pose), Salamba Bhujangasana, (Sphinx pose), Kapotasana (pigeon pose), Dharunasana (Bow pose) as well as many other such poses will help you open up your sacral chakra. An open sacral chakra has significant effects on the overall health of an individual. .

YOGA AND THE THIRD CHAKRA

It is not unusual as we run through life, to come across certain individuals who do not have the least idea what to do in life, what they feel they should be doing or who they are meant to be. The Manipura, otherwise known as the navel chakra is responsible to provide answers to these questions of an individual. This chakra is directly connected to the sense of self. Other issues like identity, self-esteem, sense of purpose, individual will and personal identity are all associated with the sacral chakra. Digestion and metabolism are physical processes also dependent on the navel chakra. A misaligned navel chakra can easily make food impossible to digest.

Yoga keeps the chakra open, balanced and aligned. This opening allows you to get in touch with your inner being, your inner will and purpose. It is not rare to find that people who practice yoga have a certain cool around them that they have achieved over time. There is no other way to explain this than the word 'peace'. This sense of peace and purpose is enough to supply anyone with the energy needed to live a life that is both challenging and exciting.

Some of the poses you may want to try in order to open up your third chakra include Kapalabhati (breath of fire), Virabhadranasa III (Warrior III), Parivrtta, Trikonasana (Triangle pose), Parsvottanasa (Pyramid pose), and many others. These different poses are aimed at opening up your chakra and aligning it with other chakras.

YOGA AND YOUR ANHATA CHAKRA

No matter the day or time, matters of the heart are as important as life itself. Be it your physical body or the quality of your life, your heart has a whole lot of say in the matter. The importance of the heart to the body can never be over explained and its importance to life is just as grave. What would you do without a beating heart? Life is too beautiful to risk going through it with a heart closed up and tired. Good thing, there is a way to heal it. The fourth chakra, which happens to be the central point of the others, is the heart chakra.

The Anhata chakra is associated with compassion and unconditional love. It is from here that you come in contact with profound truths that you may never be able to explain to anybody else. It also serves as a bridge between the lower and the upper chakras. The way you align, open and heal your heart chakra is through the practice of Yoga. The yoga poses that are directed to this chakra open the area of the chest and they help to balance the heart chakra. Poses like Camel, Standing bow pose, Cow face pose force your chest to open. The science behind it is that your heart is located in the chest region. As your chest opens up, your heart chakra is aligned.

Opening your heart chakra removes restlessness, impatience, irritability, lack of trust and lack of empathy. All of which are capable of inhibiting you from enjoying healthy relationships with others as well as with yourself. These are all possibilities that you can attain through the constant practice of the yoga poses mentioned earlier. You can begin to experience how amazing it is to give and receive empathy, trust and love.

YOGA AND THE FIFTH CHAKRA

Vishudda chakra located at the throat is the purification center. Faith, expression, inspiration and communication are all controlled here. When this chakra is balanced, you can be sure of fluent and clear thoughts, creative written and spoken expression and wisdom. Opening up your fifth chakra through yoga is important to your well-being as a person and as a body. There are various symptoms that will be visible because of the deficiencies caused by a closed chakra. Some of them include headaches, hoarseness, sore throat, neck pain, and so on.

The symptoms can go beyond the physical to include the fear of speaking, shyness, stubbornness, social anxiety, inability to express thoughts and ideas, detachment, inhibited creativity. Nobody wants to go on unable to express their deepest thoughts and emotions, no one wants to go through life without the boldness it takes to stand up for our belief, stand up to people when it is necessary and get things done when we need them to be done by others. The throat chakra has to be balanced and open to help you achieve all that. Yoga becomes very important to us because it is one very certain way of improving fluency, clarity, creativity and wisdom.

There are different yoga poses for the throat chakra. Some of these poses are Matsyasana (Fish),

Halasana (Plow), Salamba Sarvangasana (Supported Shoulderstand), King pigeon (Kapotasana), and many others. These poses allow you to stretch and exercise your neck, thyroid gland and head.

Yoga And The Sixth Chakra

Have you ever had a gut feeling about something or someone that you cannot explain? It was your third eye at work. Ajna, the sixth chakra is spectacular for perception. Often regarded as the third eye, it is responsible for controlling higher mental activities such as mental and emotional intelligence and insight. A properly aligned sixth chakra will come in handy the next time you need to make a business decision or any other important decision. A keen imagination, strong intuition and deep spiritual awareness are all resultant effects of a balanced and healthy third eye. This balance is not farfetched. You can ease yourself into it through the constant and consistent practice of yoga.

Some yoga poses that can help you activate this chakra include Child, Pyramid, Seated head to knee, side seated angle and so on.

Yoga And The Sahasrara Chakra

A certain connection with the universe is important for the individual. Have you ever felt disconnected from the entire universe? It is a feeling of despondence, lack of direction and a lack of self-understanding that results in the end. The crown chakra which happens to be the seventh helps you connect with the rest of the universe and its energy. This chakra also heightens your consciousness and pure wisdom. This is the point where the truth of the universe sits within us. Of course, you want your seventh chakra aligned, and balanced. A balanced Sahasrara results in bliss, intuitive knowledge and deeper understanding. Poses that are beneficial to your crown chakra are supported headstand, corpse pose, lotus pose, tree pose and some others.

Yoga is great for the body in a general sense, but the benefits this practice holds for the seven chakras is undeniable. If you have not added yoga to your list of frequent practices, it would be great to do that now. There is no denying the fact that yoga activates, balances, aligns and opens up your chakras.

Chapter 7.
Foods That Help
With Healing

Everyone knows that the foods you eat make a difference in the way you feel. All health specialists will tell you the same thing. However, did you know that certain foods can help to heal your chakras? They can, and it's worthwhile knowing the right kinds of foods to eat. You should also be aware that drinking sufficient water is also essential. Be mindful when you eat; chewing your food and enjoying all the tastes and textures, instead of eating on the go. Your digestive tract is the largest part of your body and if you don't give it the respect that it needs it can really give you problems – both physical and psychological. Thus, the chakras will be affected. Take your time and get used to using all of your senses actually to get more from your food. Start thinking of your food as being your friend, rather than simply the fuel you need to keep on living. There's a difference between simply living and actually optimizing your health and happiness.

You have probably heard in recent health articles about the benefits of eating brightly colored vegetables. That's certainly true when it comes to chakra healing. If you can incorporate red foods and beets into your diet, you will benefit, though don't overdo the beets as this may affect your throat chakra temporarily, taken in excess. Your root chakra is keen on spiced food, and a little tabasco sauce won't go amiss. You may even feel like your body craves this kind of taste. Learn to listen to it. It will serve you well to do so. You will also find that your root chakra enjoys lean meat, while your throat chakra is well served by a variety of fresh fruit or fruit juices. If you tend to be overweight and/or suffer from diabetes, avoid orange juice, as this concentration of fruit sugar may be detrimental to your health and fresh fruit would be a better option.

Your Solar Plexus Chakra will find its healing source in whole wheat bread, which will help in digestion. Healing can also be found in teas that are intended to calm the stomach, such as peppermint and chamomile. You may find that you enjoy eating peppermints, and rather than add the unnecessary sugar to your diet, a glass of peppermint tea is the preferred option. If you don't like drinking water, why not try adding a peppermint cordial to it, as this will also help you considerably.

Green tea is the tea of choice for the Heart Chakra, and this is particularly good for many health issues, so you won't be doing yourself a disservice introducing it as a regular drink to take the place of coffee or soda. Coffee and tea are stimulants and if you can cut down on the amount of them you drink, the better you will feel for it. The Crown chakra isn't a chakra that is affected by the foods that you eat. This is the chakra that prefers to have regular sunshine, relaxation, peace, and quiet. This chakra is calmed by meditation or relaxation exercises.

Diet in General

As a human being, you will be all too aware of your shortcomings when it comes to eating and drinking the right items. You know from normal health issues how food affects the way that you feel, but did you know how important water is to the body? Water helps to digest your food correctly, but it does much more than that. Water replenishes the body and the lost fluids that are needed for your movement and digestion. Water is especially important for those who suffer from ailments such as fibromyalgia or arthritic conditions who often forget that lack of movement and lack of water can make their situations worse. Make sure that you drink small amounts during the course of the day, which will help your chakras and will also help you to feel better.

If you know that you have been eating in excess and that this includes all of the wrong foods, one thing that can help you to detox is nettle tea. This is a wonderful way to make sure that your body keeps up its power to clean out all of the toxins that life has let get in the way.

There are many ways that you are able to work on the diet that you are taking in. Most Americans are on a diet that is not all that healthy or good for them. They are used to going out to eat all of the time, picking up something that is quick and easy at a local restaurant and using that to feed their families. This can cause a lot of bad stuff to happen to the body because all those bad nutrients, such as the sodium, the sugar, the bad fats, and the processed carbs, are all going to wreak some havoc on the body. And if the body is not able to get some of the nutrition that it needs, it is very hard for the chakras to work properly.

This means that it is time to work on making some changes to the diet that you are eating. If the description above seemed to fit into the lifestyle that you currently have, it is important to make the changes. The first changes to make is to get rid of the stuff that is so bad for the body. These are so unhealthy for the whole body and are just making you sick with all the added bad nutrients and calories.

In addition, you need to be careful about the bad sugars and sodium that are in your foods, as well as the fats and the carbs that you are taking in. Sometimes these are going to sneak their way into your diet so you need to become good at reading the labels before you purchase or make the meals for your family to eat. Watch out for some breads, some sauces, all baked goods, ice creams, French fries and more if you want to get rid of some of the bad foods that are in your diet.

Now it is time to move on to some of the foods that you should be eating to stay healthy. Here, you want to pick out foods that are healthy and whole. These are the foods that are so good for the body because they are able to provide the body with all the good nutrients that it needs, without having to put on all of the foods that are bad on the body and can make it sick. There are a few selections that you can go with including the following:

Lean meats: you will want to focus on the lean meats because they provide the body with some healthy protein that is so good for you and for helping your muscles to grow as strong as they need. While ground beef can work sometimes, but you will want to be careful because it can contain some more bad fats and cholesterol than your body needs. Lean meats like turkey, chicken, and fish are great because they provide all of the protein that the body needs without the bad stuff.

Healthy fruits and vegetables: make sure to add as many of these to your diet as you are able to each day. Fresh fruits and vegetables are so good for the body because they don't contain like any of the bad stuff that you need to worry about, they are low in calories, and you will be able to get a ton of the nutrients that you are looking for to keep the body nice and strong.

Healthy carbs: you do not have to avoid carbs all together, but you do need to be careful about the types of carbs that you are consuming. You do not want to focus on the processed and white carbs, such as those found in cheap breads or those in baked goods. These are basically going to be turned into sugars in the body which can raise your blood sugar levels and much more. Make sure that you stick with the varieties that are whole grain and will provide some added fiber and other nutrients to the diet you consume.

Low fat dairy: dairy is sometimes given a bad name, but it has a lot of the calcium that you need to keep the body nice and strong. This calcium, as well as vitamin D, can be great for the brain, the muscles, and so much more. You do need to be careful about the types of dairy that you consume. For example, if you have yogurt, you should make sure that you stick with a low fat plain yogurt and then add in fresh fruit if you would like to have that added flavor in there rather than going for the yogurt that already has the fruit inside.

In addition to making sure that you are eating the foods that you should, you will want to make sure that you are preparing the food in the proper way. You should be making these meals at home and use approved cooking methods, such as baking and steaming, rather than frying. If you are someone who is always busy and on the run, you may want to consider working with some freezer meals. With a freezer meal, you would just spend a day or two putting together some meals and then they are ready in the freezer for you any time that you need. They do take a bit of prep work to get all put together, but the convenience of being able to grab a meal when you need it rather than wasting money and harming your body is so worth it.

When you are able to follow some of the tips above about dieting and eating a diet that is full of the healthy nutrients that you need to function and feel good, you are going to notice some huge changes in your chakras. Your body will feel good, so your chakras are able to function the way that they should. Give it a try and dedicate yourself to eating foods that are healthier than ever, and you are sure to notice that your chakras will feel better in no time as well.

Exercise

If you are taking yoga classes or practicing the yoga routines that we have mentioned in this book, then you will already understand that your body responds well to this kind of treatment. Couple that with the correct breathing methods and you begin to feel happier about your state of health and welfare. Your chakras need that exercise. They need your input to unblock them, and the silly thing is that most people do not understand the power they have actually to heal their lives. Once you begin this journey, you will find that you will never go back because you enjoy being who you are and have a better understanding of what your body is asking you to do. Yoga takes an individual and teaches that individual to understand the messages he receives from his body. The mind and body work together to form the perfect harmony needed to feel good about life. Think about and exercise your senses on a regular basis, as they will serve you well. Your sense of taste, smell, sight, and hearing are all tools to be used to make your life better. Don't neglect them and remember to be mindful of their needs.

Working out is something that most people do not want to spend their time on. They are worried that it is going to be too hard, they may feel bad that they aren't able to do some of the moves that are in the program, or they just don't want to put in the work. But the great benefits that you are able to get from working out on a regular basis are amazing, and these benefits are not all centered on losing weight or toning up, although those are nice as well.

It is important to find a good workout program to start right away to help your body feel as good as possible. There are a number of different workouts that you are able to do, and to help with your health it is best to work on them all together throughout the week. If you want to do some work with the chakras, though, it seems that yoga is one of the best options that you are able to choose from. This one will help you to work on your breathing techniques, will help to align the chakras a bit more, and can help you to feel amazing in no time.

In addition to working with yoga in your life, you may want to consider doing some of the other types of exercises to help the chakras feel a bit better. Working on cardio is a great way to get the heart up and working well, and can release some of the feel good emotions and the hormones that you need to feel happy and healthy. But while a lot of people are just going to focus on the cardio that they are able to do, it is important to spend some time on strength or weight training as well. This is a great way to make those muscles nice and lean without overdoing it and this helps to burn that metabolism a bit faster and get you on the right track to feeling amazing in no time.

And of course, spending some time with stretching is critical too, if you want to avoid causing injury to the whole body. This is where yoga and other forms of stretching can come into play and will make you feel more limber and ready to take on the things that are coming up in your life.

The trick to a good workout plan is to have a lot of variety so that you are able to work out a wide variety of muscles each day while not getting bored and wanting to give up. This is why you should try to find a way to mix together the cardio, the weight training, and the stretching throughout the week, so that you can work the different muscles, not end up harming something in the process, and you can continue to have some fun while you get in that good workout. Your mind, your body, and your chakras will all thank you for this hard work.

Chapter 8.
7 Signs That Your Chakras Are Out of Balance

Weight Problems

The chakras that are affected will be the sacral chakra, solar plexus chakra, and the root chakras. Most weight problems are considered to have lifestyle, dietary, or behavioral causes, along with exercise, but one cause the most people don't consider is not being grounded. If we don't feel grounded, this is a problem with the root chakra. If the root chakra is balanced, we will feel connected to nature. It won't matter what we might be facing in life; it makes us feel secure as all our basic necessities are being met. Most of us gain weight to help us feel grounded.

We might use weight as a buffer between the world and us when our self-esteem feels off or we feel intimidated or attacked. If this is the case, our solar plexus chakra might be unbalanced. The solar plexus chakra is our center of power. It helps with confidence, self-esteem, and control.

At times we have problems feeling pleasure and getting in touch with our emotions. If we bottle up feelings about what is happening around and in us and we don't process the emotions that might have shaped our feelings about survival and self-worth, we won't experience pleasure when we eat, and our sacral chakra becomes unbalanced.

If you have a severe problem with low body weight, an intense fear of gaining any weight, and your perception about your weight is distorted, you may have been diagnosed with anorexia. People who suffer from anorexia drastically restrict how much food they eat. Bulimia is when someone eats a huge amount of food and then either takes a laxative, makes himself or herself throw up, or exercises excessively. Both of these disorders will judge a person's appearance harshly because they think they have to be severely thin to be worthy. Individuals may have trouble controlling their own self-image because they think they have physical flaws. Both of these disorders are caused by an unbalanced solar plexus.

Mental Disorders

Anxiety: All of the chakras can be affected. It all depends on the type of anxiety you are experiencing. Anxiety is a part of our daily lives. When we get an intense, persistent, or excessive worry that takes over our existence, it is totally debilitating. If you suffer from anxiety, it could turn into terror or fear in minutes and, thus, turn anxiety into a panic attack. It can also mess up our quality of life.

It all depends on the type of anxiety you have, but it could affect any one of the chakras that are involved. If the crown chakra is out of balance, we might feel as if we aren't connected to the God, Goddess, Universe, Source, or Divine. If our anxiety is from the third eye being out of balance, we feel anxious about the unknown and we don't trust our intuition.

You might feel anxious about saying how you actually feel, expressing yourself, and communicating with others if your throat chakra is not balanced. If are feeling intimidated, pressure to do well, completely overwhelmed by everything, or caught in a power struggle within a relationship, your solar plexus chakra is out of balance. If your sacral chakra is out of balance, you will have feelings of shame or guilt due to emotions that are so intense that you have not processed them completely. This can happen because of past traumas like sexual abuse. If we feel anxious about our surviving in this world like money, shelter, food, etc., the root chakra is not balanced. This makes us feel as if we are in a constant survival mode.

Depression: The chakras that are affected are the heart and crown chakras. Depression happens for many reasons. It might pass through temporarily at times. At other times, it could be a presence in our lives that never goes away. For people who suffer from depression, it could be debilitating. Depression might feel like constant hopelessness, emptiness, or sadness. You might not have any pleasure in your daily activities and feel like life isn't worth living. It might affect your sleep or appetite, causing you to sleep too much or not sleep at all. You might even have thought about suicide or death.

When you are depressed, you will have a deep-seated feeling of loneliness. If you feel connected to the world and the Universe, the crown chakra is balanced and open. If you feel angry toward the Universe about your life, this shows your energy is out of harmony. Having an unbalanced heart chakra might cause depression because we aren't connected to ourselves.

Panic Attacks: The chakras that are affected are the root, solar plexus, and heart chakras. Panic attacks happen when we are struck with disabling, acute, and sudden anxiety. These can be accompanied by feelings of impending doom, shortness of breath, shaking, trembling, sweating, increased heart rate, pounding heart, and palpitations. These attacks can happen if we aren't connected to our heart chakra and don't listen to what it is telling us. The root chakra gets involved when fear and panic set in since our fear for survival gets triggered. If our heart chakra feels disconnected and we are in a constant state of fear, the solar plexus feels as if we have been punched in the stomach since our confidence and self-esteem live here.

Cancer

All the chakras are affected by this horrible disease. Cancer happens when cells that are abnormal get created and divide at an uncontrollable rate. They infiltrate and destroy good body tissue. This can happen on many levels and symptoms can vary depending on the part of the body that gets affected. Symptoms might include thick areas under the skin, palpable lumps, skin changes, weight changes, fatigue, and many others. Factors that can increase the risk of cancer can include environment, health conditions, family history, habits, and age. The Mayo Clinic has stated that most cancers happen in people who don't have any known risk factors. Cancer could be the result of deep hurt and resentment that has not been processed, denied, or ignored. It can manifest in toxic emotions, grief, or hatred that eats away at us.

These manifest on several levels because of a result of having an imbalance in certain chakras:

- Cancers of esophagus, larynx, and thyroid: Throat chakra

- Lung cancer: Heart and throat chakras

- Brain tumors: Crown chakra

- Rectal and prostate cancer: Root and sacral chakra

- Cancers of rectum, colon, uterus, ovaries, and cervix: Sacral chakra

- Cancers of the pancreas, intestines, liver, and stomach: Solar plexus chakra

- Breast cancer: Heart chakra

Headaches

The chakras that are affected by this are the crown and third eye chakras. If you get headaches that aren't caused by physical imbalances, it might be an indication that one of your chakras is unbalanced. If you have a headache in the front that includes symptoms of pressure behind the eyes or sinus pressure, this is usually disharmony in the third eye.

This type of headache might indicate that you have been focusing on your intelligence and you fear your spirituality. You can only see the reality in life, and you don't trust your intuition. When these headaches happen, it is because you are ignoring the inner wisdom that you possess. If you get "hints" but never act on them, you aren't honoring your third eye's wisdom. You might feel like you need to pursue new opportunities, but you don't do so. You might also experience a knowing that a specific person might be ill and won't feel like being around others. You engage them anyway. Opposing intuitive hints could cause imbalance and discord with the third eye chakra.

If you have a headache on the top of your head in the center, it might be from an imbalance in the crown chakra. This might mean you have a hard time trusting your life path, or seeing the larger picture, or even finding faith in yourself and your connection to the Divine. You might also feel unsatisfied or alone.

Reproductive Issues

Infertility: The chakras that are affected by this will be the solar plexus, root, and sacral chakras. If a woman can't conceive a child after many attempts for over one year, this is called infertility. Many will experience infertility, but the fear, and frustration that the woman experiences creates a lot of stress and possibly shame. The sacral chakra is the one that is affected because it is associated with the genitals and womb and because it is the seat of all emotions. Most people who deal with infertility battle with many severe emotions. It makes them wonder, "Am I making the right decision?" "Do I even want to be a parent?" "Do I have the right partner?" "I might not even be a good parent." "How is this going to change my life?"

There could be physical causes like high follicle-stimulating hormone, lack of menstruation, low sperm count, poor egg quality, and other issues could be to blame. Most of the time, there is a high stress level for the people who are trying to conceive. Since infertility can trigger family issues, the root chakra is involved, too. For people who are trying to conceive, added difficulty can develop if they are trying to have a family and aren't getting any support from a significant other. They might also be worried about passing on undesirable traits to their children. Making a new life is a challenge to a person's self-esteem, it can make them feel powerless and this becomes a solar plexus issue since this is our power center.

Uterine Cysts and Fibroids: The chakra that is affected is the sacral chakra. The Mayo Clinic states that uterine fibroids are growths that are in the uterus that aren't cancerous. They often happen during childbearing years. A lot of women may experience uterine fibroids sometime in their lives. Most of the time, they don't cause any symptoms but for others, they can grow to a large size and cause pain during menstruation, when having a bowel movement, or when you are digesting food. They can cause problems in breathing.

Cysts are sacs filled with fluid that are located on the ovaries. If there is a growth inside the uterus, it might be a sign that the sacral chakra is not balanced. There is an actual block to the reproductive area. The energy is telling you that there is a blocked energy flow inside. You might be holding onto toxic, negative, and old thoughts, feelings, or emotions that are attempting to flow energy into dead ends. This could include relationships or jobs that you have outgrown or conflict with your relationships, reproduction, abundance, or creativity.

Joint Pain

Hip Pain: If you have problems with your hips that aren't caused by any physical trauma, there is usually a sacral chakra problem. Our hips hold onto a lot of unexpressed emotions that haven't been dealt with and that we keep avoiding. Since the sacral chakra is the seat of our emotions, we could cause an imbalance if we don't honor our feeling.

Leg Pain: The chakras that are affected will be the solar plexus or root chakra. Leg pain is usually linked to an imbalance in the root chakra. Leg pain might symbolize a resistance to moving forward in life. This could manifest in self-sabotaging behaviors that are based on fear, for example, a fear of failure or fear that we might not get what we want. If this is the case, the root chakra could be linked to the solar plexus chakra and both are out of balance. It is mainly a root chakra problem because of fear about clothing, water, food, housing, or bills.

Neck Pain: The chakra that is affected here is the throat chakra. If the neck pain hasn't been caused by any physical trauma, it could be that your throat chakra is out of balance due to the way you are interacting with the world. If you don't express yourself honestly and openly or if you try to hide specific parts of yourself like insecurities or fears from others, it can create imbalances to the throat chakra. There are many reasons why you might hold yourself back, but the end result is always the same: neck pain.

Sciatica: The chakra that is affected by this is the sacral and root chakras. Sciatica is pain that goes from the lower back down through the hips, buttocks, and down each leg. If it isn't caused by trauma, sciatic pain could mean a root chakra that is out of balance. This chakra deals with problems regarding your being and survival. If a primal problem comes up in your life: fear that your basic necessities will be taken away, whether or not you can provide for your children, how you will pay your bills, or if you be able to eat today, this means your root chakra is out of balance. Sciatica usually symbolizes your fear about the future and money. At times, if you have sciatic pain, it could mean you don't feel safe.

Back Pain: If you have pain anywhere in the back that wasn't caused by physical trauma, it might be telling you about your chakra health. Pain could range from a dull ache that makes your back tight to a sharp acute pain that hinders your range of motion.

Upper Back: The chakras that are affected are the heart and throat chakras. If you don't speak the truth or if you experience heartbreak, threats to loving yourselves or problems loving others, the tension could manifest as pain or tension in the upper back. You might feel as if you are holding back love, unloved, or unsupported.

Middle Back: The chakras that are affected are the solar plexus and heart chakras. Everyone has issues about love, holding onto hurts from the past, our power being challenged, or feeling loved, you might feel pain or tension in the middle part of your back. This might happen if you get stuck in those feelings from the past and might become filled with guilt over things you said or done.

Lower Back: The chakras that are affected are the root and sacral chakras. If you are feeling challenged in creative expression, relationships, or abundance, you might feel pain and tension in your lower back. Holding these emotions back or just not processing them and having problems with survival and getting your basic needs met might mean pain for your back.

Asthma and Allergies

The chakra that is affected is the heart chakra. If you experience narrow airways and are producing excess mucous, it could trigger shortness of breath, wheezing, and coughing. If you have allergies, your immune system will make antibodies that recognize a certain allergen is harmful, even if it isn't. Both of these conditions cause problems with one's daily life. Sometimes these conditions can be caused by a compromised immune system and might cause inflammation of your digestive system, sinuses, airway, or skin. It could also cause respiratory distress. Since these are in the heart chakra, such reactions might mean that this chakra is out of balance, especially if you have problems with compassion, love, heartache, and grief.

Chapter 9.
Chakras, Endocrine System And The Immune System

In addition to the benefits mentioned earlier, there are many things that chakras control including the efficient functioning of our endocrine system and our emotions. Let us look at each in a bit of detail:

Let us start by recalling the 7 primary chakras and their locations:

Root Chakra – situated at the base of the spine

Sacral Chakra – situated below the navel

Solar Plexus Chakra – situated above the navel

<u>Heart Chakra</u> – situated in the middle of the chest

<u>Throat Chakra</u> – situated in the throat

<u>Third Eye Chakra</u> – situated at the center of the forehead

<u>Crown Chakra</u> – situated at the top of the head

The Endocrine System

Next, let us look at the Endocrine System in our body. The Endocrine System is our body's central mechanism of control. It consists of many ductless glands that are responsible for secreting, producing, and distributing different kinds of hormones required for various physiological functions of our body.

These hormones are directly sent through the bloodstream to the places that need them. Effective functioning of the Endocrine System is essential for overall good physical and mental health. The Endocrine System consists of the following elements:

The Pineal Gland – The most important hormone secreted by this gland is melatonin that is responsible for maintaining and regulating your body's circadian rhythm or the internal biological clock. This cone-shaped gland along with the pituitary gland regulates and balances the entire biological and glandular functioning in our body. The third eye chakra can be activated optimally when the pineal and the pituitary glands work perfectly in tandem.

The Pituitary Gland – Also referred to as the 'master gland,' the pituitary gland controls the activities and functioning of most other glands. Attached to the hypothalamus (between the eyes), the pituitary gland regulates the functioning of other organs and other glands. It communicates via signals in different forms.

This pea-shaped gland works in tandem with the pineal gland controls and balances the overall smooth functioning of our body's physiological and biological activities. The energy of the third eye chakra can be released when these two glands are well synchronized with each other.

Pancreas – The two kinds of hormones produced by the pancreas are needed for two basic functions; one to aid in digestion and the other to control energy levels in our body.

Ovaries – These glands produce the female hormones namely progesterone and estrogen and also produce and release eggs for reproduction

Testes – These glands come in pairs and are responsible for the production and release of the male hormone, testosterone. They also produce and release sperms.

Thyroid – A very important gland, the thyroid is responsible for regulating the heart rate, the metabolic rate and also controls a few digestive functions along with bone maintenance, muscle control, and brain development. The thyroxin produced by the thyroid controls the rate at which our body converts stored food into energy for use. A malfunctioning thyroid can be quite a debilitating factor that comes in the way of a leading a happy life for anyone.

Parathyroid – This gland controls calcium levels in the bloodstream so that the muscles and the nerves function smoothly. The parathyroid also helps in keeping bones healthy and strong.

Hypothalamus – This gland responds to multiple external and internal factors and triggers various reactions to enable stability and a consistent state in our body. The hypothalamus triggers various physiological reactions in response to feelings of hunger, the temperature of your body, feelings of excessive eating, blood pressure, and others. Based on these conditions, it sends signals to other glands and organs to respond appropriately to these triggers to enable a stable and consistent condition of your body.

Adrenal Glands – These glands secrete different kinds of hormones referred to as 'chemical messengers' which travel through the bloodstream to triggers physiological and chemical reactions in various organs.

The Immune System

Millions and millions of cells come together and waltz together in perfect harmony exchanging critical information thereby triggering appropriate and important physiological, biological, and chemical reactions in our body. The cells of the immune system help organs and organ systems in our body to function smoothly helping us live a happy and peaceful life.

Moreover, those cells that are not performing optimally are retired and new ones are automatically generated to take their place thereby enhancing our health and our longevity. If these weak cells are not correctly replaced in the immune system, they end up sending erroneous signals to all parts of the body resulting in disorders and discomforts such as weak digestion, general body weakness and delayed recovery from even simple illnesses.

The way modern medicines work to set this right is by suppressing the action of the well-functioning cells too until such time all the cells do not achieve the same level of functioning. The medication is continued until all the cells in the immune system get back into the synchronized dancing pattern. This is where chakra healing can help in getting our immune system in order.

The Thymus Gland – It plays an important role in the production of T-cells which form an essential part of the white blood cells that form the core of our immune system. In fact, if you speak to any chakra healer, he or she will tell you the dance of the immune system is the most beautiful and well-coordinated dance in our body.

Chakras And Glands

If you notice the locations of the glands, you will see that they are more or less placed close to different chakras. Although the traditional systems do not speak about the connection between chakras and glands, the modern followers and experts started outlining clear connections between the various chakras, glands, organs and the immune system of the body.

Each chakra is connected to different glands of the endocrine system and facilitates the smooth functioning of that particular gland. Here is a list of the various chakras, the glands they regulate, their functions and the signs of warnings associated with an inefficiently functioning gland/chakra:

Root Chakra – This is connected to the adrenal glands and stands for self-preservation and physical energy. The issues that the root chakra and the adrenal glands handle are associated with survival and security. In the males, the sacral chakra is closely linked to the gonads. The fight/flight response of the adrenal glands located at the top of the kidneys is directly connected to the survival drive of the root chakra.

A weak root chakra could result in a weakened metabolism and immune system resulting from a compromised working of the adrenal glands which are responsible for releasing and producing chemical messengers needed for all the physiological, chemical and biological functions of your body.

A not-so-strong root chakra results in nervousness and a sense of insecurity whereas an overly working root chakra could result in greed and a sense of excessive materialism.

Sacral Chakra – Governs the reproductive glands which are the ovaries (for the females) and the testes (for the males. The well-balanced and healthy root chakra facilitates the uninterrupted functioning of these glands ensuring well-developed sexuality in the person.

The root chakra also regulates the production and secretion of the sex hormones. The potential for life formation in the ovaries is reflected in the sacral chakra as these two energies are connected.

When this chakra is open and free, you are able to express your sexuality well without being overly emotional. You feel a comforting sense of intimacy with your partner. A healthy sacral chakra enhances your passion and liveliness and helps you manage your sexuality without feeling burdened with undue emotions.

A sacral chakra that is not functioning at its peak efficiency is bound to leave you frigid, very close to people and relationships, and poker-faced. On the contrary, a weak sacral chakra will make you feel overly and unnecessarily, emotionally compelling you to attach yourself to people for a sense of security and belonging. Your feelings could be overly sexual towards one and all.

Solar Plexus Chakra – This controls the pancreas, which is directly connected to the sugar (through the control of insulin secretion) and, therefore, energy levels in your body. Thus, if this chakra is not working properly you could potentially have a weak pancreas, resulting in a compromised metabolic state. Compromised pancreas could lead to digestive problems, lowered blood sugar levels, ulcers, poor memory, etc. which are all connected with a bad metabolism.

Heart Chakra – Regulates the thymus gland and through it, the entire immune system. Being the center of love, compassion, spirituality, and group consciousness, a malfunctioning heart chakra will result in the malfunctioning of the thymus gland leaving you prone to low immunity.

Our feelings and thoughts towards ourselves play a crucial role in keeping our immune system working well. When we love ourselves our immune system is powerful and strong. When we are uncertain of ourselves and our strengths and our capabilities, we feel disappointed which drives us to react wrongly to negative things.

All these negativities leave our immune system weak and we end up holding on to toxins. It is imperative to keep our heart chakra healthy by investing time and energy in self-love so that our immune system is strengthened. An underactive heart chakra makes you feel distant and cold and an overactive one could result in selfish love in your heart. Be wary of both states and work at keeping your chakra balanced.

Throat Chakra – controls and regulates the thyroid gland and hence is directly responsible for a healthy metabolism and to regulate body temperature. This is the center of communication and plays a vital role in the way you speak, write, or think. An unbalanced throat chakra results in a malfunctioning thyroid resulting in an overall poor physical, mental, and emotional health.

Third Eye Chakra – directly controls the functioning of the pituitary gland or the master gland which controls and regulates other organs and glands in the human body. The Pineal gland is many times associated with this chakra too, as we already know that a well-coordinated, combined working of the pineal and the pituitary glands is responsible to keep our entire body, mind, and spirit well-oiled and working well.

Crown Chakra – This regulates the functioning of the pineal gland, which controls our biological cycle and our circadian rhythm.

Connection Between Glands And Chakras

Even the slightest disturbances in the chakras or our energy centers can result in physical manifestations of issues and problems. When the chakras don't function efficiently the corresponding glands and organs they are associated with are also affected.

Chakras as you already know are the energy centers in our body and have no physiological or physical shape or form. These energy centers influence the way we live in different layers of our lives, including the biological, the physical, the emotional, and the psychic layers.

When any of the energy centers malfunction or become imbalanced, the problems are manifested in a physical, mental, or spiritual form. An underactive or an overactive chakra can cause problems for you. Keeping them balanced is critical for your overall health.

Any disturbance even in one energy center could result in problems in any other chakra and/or related glands and organs. For example, if there is a blockage in the heart chakra, you are going to feel unloved or listless or could have high blood pressure etc. All these problems could affect other organs which, in turn, can potentially harm associated chakras.

Therefore, it is imperative to keep all chakras in perfect balance to achieve overall physical, emotional, and spiritual health for yourself. Let us look at some examples of how a malfunctioning of chakras can affect the associated gland.

The Third Eye Chakra And The Pituitary And The Pineal Glands

When the third eye chakra is imbalanced or not working at its peak of efficiency, the functioning of both the pineal and pituitary glands will be affected leading to associated problems. For example, the pituitary is the master gland that regulates the functioning of other glands. So, when the third eye chakra is inefficient, other glands can also be affected negatively resulting in an overall breakdown of your systems.

The pituitary gland regulates intellect and emotion and working in conjunction with the pineal gland helps achieve overall balance in your body. The pineal gland will either resonate or counter the effects of pituitary gland for optimum benefit to our body and mind. Therefore, the third eye chakra is required to be given a lot of importance during your chakra healing and maintenance process.

The Heart Chakra And The Thymus Gland

Located in the middle of your chest, the heart chakra or the anahata controls and regulates the working of the thymus gland which is an important aspect of our immune system. A calm and balanced heart chakra results in an effectively-working nervous system and prevents undue agitation of your mind.

Here is a simple technique to help connect and activate your thymus gland. Tap gently in the middle of your chest at the collarbone level with your fingers. This helps in calming down agitated nerves. When you gently tap at the collar level about 3-4 inches away on each side helps to increase your energy levels.

Glands And Chakra Healing

Chakra healing will lead to improved functioning of the endocrine system which is great for physical healing of your body. The connection between glands and chakras represent a link between the energy points in your body to the physiological and physical functions.

Another useful entry point for chakra healing is the nervous system which is connected to glands and organs in multiple ways and at multiple points. A chakra healing session is ideally begun by calming the nerves and then targeting a particular gland and/or chakra.

By understanding the connection between chakras and the glands, you can use healing in different ways that will help you overcome physical, emotional, mental, and spiritual issues in your body and mind. Connecting the chakras and the glands will help in your overall well-being.

Chapter 10.
The Science Behind Chakras

When you hear talk about chakras the first thing you associate them with is probably spirituality. After all, the concept of chakras has its roots in ancient India, the very personification of spirituality if there ever was one! From Hindu gods and goddesses to the origins of Buddhism, ancient India covers a wider spectrum of spirituality and religious tradition than just about any other place or culture on the face of the Earth. Modern-day forms of meditation and yoga owe their very existence to the mystics and healers of the subcontinent. Therefore, it is no wonder that the tradition of chakras evokes such a rich and reverent sense of spirituality. However, there is another side to chakras, one which is more modern and certainly less spiritual, at least at face value. This other side is the science behind chakras.

Modern science has produced countless discoveries in terms of the human body and the role that energy plays in our very existence. While the concept of energy is certainly nothing new, the quantification of energy definitely is. Never before have we been able to actually see and measure the amounts of energy being generated by a living thing. With today's science and technology such feats are now commonplace. In fact, much of modern medicine utilizes the ability to measure and monitor the energy levels within the human body, thus determining the health and wellbeing of an individual in ways that the ancient mystics of India would have doubtlessly understood all too well. After all, the idea that energy makes up all living things is something we might consider revolutionary in scientific terms, but it is very old news to those who have been practicing chakra health and wellbeing. Indeed, the knowledge that we have obtained through modern breakthroughs in technology has done little more than validating the ancient traditions of chakra energy and their role in human life.

One of the first things to recognize when it comes to the science behind chakras is the significance of just where the chakras are located. Placing the energy centers of the subtle body along a central axis makes good sense as they are more balanced and centered along that line. However, you could ask why chakras weren't placed below the Root Chakra position, at the knees or feet for example. Alternatively, you could question why chakras were not allocated to the hands. After all, what part of the body is more associated with energy than the hands or the feet? Yet the seven main chakras are contained within a short span, traveling up the central axis of the human body along the spinal column. And here is where the science behind chakras begins to take shape. It turns out that the spinal column is, in fact, the conduit through which electrical impulses are transmitted from the brain to all other parts of the body. The nerves which run through the spinal column are virtual telephone lines, bringing every sort of message from the command center of the brain to all other parts of the physical body. Thus, the spinal column is nothing short of an energy highway, seeing energy flow from the brain to the body and from the body back to the brain again.

The fact that the spinal column is the path for energy to flow throughout the body would be enough to get anyone to consider the validity of the chakras, regardless of their spiritual beliefs. However, this is not the end of the story. What is even more striking is that the locations of the lower five chakras correspond directly to actual nerve clusters along the spinal column. This means that not only did the ancients understand the function of the spinal column, but they also were aware of the significance of the nerve clusters along it! Just as the chakras are considered energy centers of the subtle body, the nerve clusters along the spinal column, five in total, are actually energy centers of the physical body. Some might argue that this is nothing spectacular. After all, if anyone studied a dissected body, they would see the nerve centers in the spinal column. While this is true, it must be understood that those same ancients had no modern equipment with which to measure the energy in those nerve centers. Thus, those nerves could have served any function to the casual observer. Yet the ancient Indian sages knew somehow that those bundles of nerves were, in fact, the centers of energy in the physical human body.

Perhaps this is a classic matter of which came first, the chicken or the egg? While it is possible that the ancients studied the anatomy of the body, it is also entirely feasible that their knowledge of the chakras had little or nothing to do with their understanding of the human body. We may never know what inspired their belief in seven separate energy centers along a central axis, but what we can be sure of is that their knowledge goes hand in hand with the knowledge we are only now beginning to acquire regarding how the physical body works. It is therefore entirely possible that the ancients were made aware of the workings of the subtle body and that only now can we see the direct correlation between our subtle form and our physical form. Either way, modern science, and medicine have only served to validate the concept that energy centers do in fact exist along the spinal column, and that the health and wellbeing of these centers greatly impact our overall physical health and wellbeing.

The five nerve clusters along the spinal column account for the first five chakras, beginning with the Root Chakra and ending with the Throat Chakra. While the Third Eye Chakra and the Crown Chakra are not located in the spinal column itself they still follow the same central axis. There are a few theories regarding the scientific nature of these two chakras, and it is worth examining two of the main ones. First, there is the theory that the sixth and seventh chakras are related to the pineal and the pituitary glands. In the case of the sixth or the Third Eye Chakra, the pineal gland is seen as the corresponding energy center. The significance of this is that the pineal gland is responsible for creating melatonin which regulates sleep patterns. Since the third eye is considered the subconscious mind in many traditions it is profoundly significant that the Third Eye Chakra would be located in a place where sleep, and thus dreams are regulated. Many ancient traditions view dreams as the realm of the subconscious, equally real and important to physical reality. The idea that the ancients placed the seat of the intellect and subconscious mind in the same vicinity as the pineal gland has to be far more than mere coincidence.

Physicians and philosophers alike have attributed the pineal gland with such things as the intellect and even the soul itself. René Descartes was a world-renowned scientist and philosopher in the sixteen hundreds. He wrote several books on anatomy and the soul, two of which dealt with the pineal gland in particular. According to Descartes, the pineal gland was where our soul resided and was the very place where all thoughts originated. While modern science is still struggling to understand the complexities of the human brain it might be time to consider the patterns already emerging. The fact that the pineal gland is responsible for sleep, and thus dreams, and that some prominent thinkers have attributed it to the center of thought and the subconscious self, coupled with the fact that the Third Eye Chakra is located in the same region, should be enough to convince anyone that these assertions are in fact true. Again, this is just one more example of where the physical body closely mirrors the dynamics of the subtle body.

The Crown Chakra, or the seventh chakra, is the highest chakra of the seven. Located at the crown of the head, it resides between the physical body and the realm beyond. One theory links this chakra with the pituitary gland, which makes a lot of sense when you understand the functions of the pituitary gland.

The main function of the pituitary gland is to produce and secrete hormones—chemicals that affect functions throughout the rest of the body. Some of the functions affected by the hormones produced by the pituitary gland include Thyroid function, water absorption, and regulation of temperature, pain and pain relief, regulation of blood pressure, growth, and sex organ functions. All in all, the pituitary gland can be seen as a controller of just about every facet of the physical body's function and wellbeing. In a way, the pituitary gland is like the conductor of an orchestra, overseeing that every member of the orchestra performs their part exactly as it ought to be performed. Is it any wonder that this is where the chakra associated with a higher being is located? After all, what function does the Higher Being have than to oversee and regulate the function of all life? Again, is its mere coincidence that the chakra centers have been placed where they have, or is modern science simply revealing that the wisdom of the ancients is, in fact, accurate and deserves greater attention and respect?

The association of the sixth and seventh chakras with the pineal and pituitary glands is just one theory which serves to confirm the validity of the chakra tradition. Another theory which deserves attention is the one that focuses on the general regions of the Third Eye and Crown Chakras. This theory doesn't focus on specific glands, but rather it focuses on the area of the brain and the top of the head. In the case of the sixth or Third Eye Chakra, the location of this chakra is basically in the forehead region, which is where the brain itself is largely located. Again, this has great significance as the brain is scientifically known to be the seat of all thought, emotions and even dreams, thus it can be considered the seat of the subconscious. While this is nothing new in terms of our understanding of the human condition, it should be noted that different cultures throughout history viewed things quite differently. The ancient Greeks, for example, saw various organs as the seat of the soul, including the heart, liver and even the abdomen. In fact, the Greeks believed that the lower organs were the originators of emotional joy and or pain.

That said, the notion that the brain is the center of thought, creativity, and even the subconscious is, in fact, a very recent one. Only within the last few hundred years has the seat of the mind found its way to the head. Thus, the fact that the ancient Indian sages placed the chakra responsible for intellect and wisdom in the forehead was far more than mere luck. Again, due to the primitive science and technology available at the time it is hard to imagine that the placement of the Third Eye Chakra had anything to do with a deeper understanding of human anatomy and physiology. Rather, it seems that by understanding the workings and design of a person's subtle body the ancients were able to lay the foundations for a more accurate and in-depth understanding of the workings and design of the physical body.

The Crown Chakra is a bit of a mystery in terms of its location on the human body. Depending on the tradition you read, this chakra is located at or just above the crown of a person's head. In terms of spiritual significance, this makes perfect sense as the Crown Chakra is literally your connection to the higher realm of spirit. In a sense you could relate the Crown Chakra to the leaves on a tree, existing between the tree itself and the air all around it. And, just as the leaves of a tree absorb the energy from the air and the sun, so too, the Crown Chakra absorbs the energy from the higher realms. Still, this doesn't really do much for proving that the ancients had some advanced understanding of how the physical body worked as a result of their insights regarding the subtle body. That is unless you consider a concept that is gaining more and more acceptance within the scientific community. This concept is the one regarding auras. The aura of a person is literally an envelope of energy that radiates from and surrounds the person. Recent advances in photographic and electromagnetic technology have enabled us to actually see the human aura for the first time in recorded history. And this phenomenon has gone a long way to changing our understanding of how energy affects life overall.

While a person's aura envelops their whole body, the most visible elements of it are around the head. Thus, the virtual energy of a person can be seen just above their shoulders and above the crown of their head. This is where the ancient symbol of the halo comes to mind. When we think of a halo we are reminded of the holiest people, or angels or deities themselves. Additionally, while halos are normally associated with Christianity, the fact of the matter is that they have representations throughout many traditions across many different times and places throughout history. Thus, while the traditions themselves may differ, the association of halos with purity or divinity remains constant. Furthermore, the more divine or holy a person was, the larger and brighter their halo was. Suddenly we have our physical connection with the location of the seventh chakra. The Crown Chakra—that which connects a person with the divine, is in the same place as the energy 'crown' of a person's physical body. And, just as this energy crown lingers on and just above the head, so too the Crown Chakra does the same. Due to the realization that our physical body has an energy envelope of sorts, our representation of the human form may have to be changed from its current physical only form to one which incorporates its energy aspect as well.

The fact that modern science has discovered energy centers in the same locations as for where the ancients placed the seven main chakras is nothing short of extraordinary. Even the harshest skeptic would have to take a moment to consider the significance of what this actually means. However, in case you thought that this was the only correlation between the chakra traditions and modern science, rest assured, there is more! The chakras and the nerve centers are described as focal points for energy. This energy was seen as the electrical communications between the brain and the body and nothing more for many years. However, modern breakthroughs in the fields of electromagnetism and quantum physics have led to yet more correlations between modern science and ancient wisdom. Modern research has begun to determine that not all energy is the same. Just as radio waves exist on different frequencies, so too, energy can exist in different forms. The variations of energy are often referred to in terms of vibrations. Lower vibrations create different forms of energy than higher vibrations. In fact, it is theorized that matter itself is merely energy on a really low vibrational frequency. This is the basis of all teleportation theories. Converting matter to energy is not as difficult as it once seemed since matter itself is now seen as a level of energy. Still, how does this relate to chakras? Simply put, science is now realizing that the human body does, in fact, absorb energy from its surroundings as well as from the food that it ingests.

Once science realized that electromagnetic energy is all around us, moving past us and even through us at all times, the question was raised as to how this energy affected us. On the physiological level, certain energies can, in fact, be dangerous. People who live or work near areas with high electromagnetic activity often contract cancers and other ailments, now being linked to the high concentrations of energy. There has also been an association of energy and mood, suggesting that a person's mind can be directly influenced by the energy in the environment. At first, this doesn't make sense since energy, like radio waves, needs a receiver in order to be of any actual value. And, just like a radio, the human body would need to convert the energy received into usable information. Simply receiving the radio waves is not enough for a radio to play music. A radio must convert those radio waves back into vibrations in order to produce the appropriate sounds. Here we find two distinct correlations to chakra energy and wellbeing.

The first correlation is in terms of the chakras acting as energy centers. By understanding that energy flows around us and through us at all times, these centers take on a whole new meaning. Not only do they generate energy that flows through our physical and subtle bodies, affecting our overall health and wellbeing, but they also receive energy from the environment. This means that they absorb as well as generate energy. Thus, when a chakra is closed or damaged its ability to absorb useful energy is significantly reduced. This is like not being able to digest food properly. It is no wonder, in light of this, that damaged chakras can so significantly reduce a person's health and wellbeing. The importance of having healthy, vibrant chakras is therefore even more critical as the health of our chakras determines our ability to take in energy.

Chapter 11.
Things to Avoid

We can all get a little carried away in a practice or a process. We can get lazy and not put in as much effort as we should. There are always fluctuations with life because we need to be flexible when the unexpected occurs. When you are going through a chakra awakening experience it will be very 'eye-opening' and transformative. As a lot of people are discovering these tools and methods and choosing to align with higher consciousness, there are several reports available of what many people have encountered in their own experiences.

For a lot of us, it is an amazing and powerful shift and rediscovery that can turn your life upside down and help you to work on the life path and goals you are actually wishing for, rather than living the life you thought you had to for whatever reasons. Using your intuition to guide you along the way can help, but it won't always be accessible and here's why: when you are in an awakening experience, you are dealing with your past and your present problems so that you can invest in a greater future.

Your processing experience is what will have to happen in order for you to be able to live in value to your chakra energies. What this means is that you will have to enjoy the turmoil of poking your internal hornet's nest, so to speak. Whatever you are going through right now, today has likely had a connection to the energy of your past that has been locked into your 7 chakras. In order to find your way into a new balance, you will have to see, know, feel and sense things that might have caused you pain in the past that are presently manifesting as other issues, like chronic pain, chronic fatigue syndrome, hormone imbalances, depression or anxiety, and so on.

There are ways that you can help yourself have a smoother, lighter, and more carefree and joyful journey as you stimulate the negative energies that you are working to let go of and purge. Troubleshooting chakra awakening is a part of the process that will help you to stay grounded and putting your best intentions and focus on healing.

The following list provides you with some key points about what you should avoid or be aware of as you go through the purging and cleansing experience.

- Avoid processed foods, as well as high sugar content foods and drinks, alcohol, and drugs. All of these chemicals have a powerful interaction with your energy and your vital organ systems. If you actually want to heal your chakras and your whole body, then you may have to make some significant changes in your diet and nutrition.

- Avoid attitudes and behaviors that will perpetuate bad habits and negativity. Seek to have a more positive outlook and be open to letting go of patterns that cause you to feel unhealthy.

- Avoid situations, people and environments that feel 'toxic' to you. There are a lot of scenarios that are unhealthy for people and sometimes we just go along with it because we feel like we have to. Part of stimulating a healing process and purging the negativity in our bodies is the letting go of particular people, places or activities that keep us feeling 'off' in our world.

- Avoid participating in anything that causes you physical or emotional harm or pain. Some events in life are unavoidable and we cannot control everything, but we can control some things and if you are repeatedly offering yourself something painful, it will cost your healing journey and cause it to take a lot longer.

- Avoid extremes. Extremes could be anything like binge-watching television for several days in a row, to drinking to excess, to uprooting and changing your job or living situation out of nowhere. These things may be tempting and are often coping mechanisms when we are uncomfortable with our awakening experiences. Looking for healthier ways to process is a much better action for the chakras.

- Process your opening with a healthy diet, sleep practice, hydration, and quality of life that will feel supportive and compatible with how you are going through your chakra awakening.

- Explore alternative methods for health care, like yoga, acupuncture, Reiki, massage, lymphatic drainage, sound baths, and deprivation tanks. All of these methods are ways that you can connect more deeply to the process of helping your chakra energy shift and heal. Self-care is a huge problem in our culture; most people have not learned how to make it a regular part of everyday life.

- Arrange for space to be alone and have quiet, reflective moments. It doesn't have to be a meditation or a specific practice; it can simply be having solitude and journaling or contemplating what your present feelings or state of mind is.

- Develop daily routines and habits that support your chakra awakening and healing journey.

You don't have to do everything all at once; that would be too extreme. Start slowly and change one thing at a time to include more healthy energy healing practices.

- Be patient and kind to yourself. This awakening experience is about you and your life and how you want to live well. It can be easy to go overboard and feel unhappy with your progress, or like you aren't doing enough. That kind of belief or attitude will just cause even more negative energy for you to release, purge and heal, and so it is best to help yourself feel well along the journey.

All of these types of things can take time to find balance with and incorporate into a new lifestyle and routine. It's never easy to just change everything all at once and that is why it is best to plan for a long road to travel and that as you slowly start making some changes your chakras will start to change with you.

One of the biggest issues that we all have in our modern age is instant gratification. Everyone wants a miracle cure, or easy fix to a lot of problems or life issues and the number one way that people fall off the chakra awakening wagon is to give up and stay with their lower vibrational energy because it is easy, familiar, and it doesn't require any hard work.

Awakening your chakras isn't hard, especially if you are wanting to create a more balanced and healthy life. It can actually be a joyful and pleasurable experience for a person to experience and as long as you have that attitude about it going in, you are likely to have a much better time hanging in there when things feel a little rough around the edges.

One major aspect of this practice is that you will have to go over it on a daily or regular basis in order to make the really big, positive changes and shifts. If you are not ready to make that a part of your life habits, then you may need more time to do some research and mentally prepare for the possibilities of making so much change in your life.

So, here are some additional tips to help you stay focused and avoid issues that may come up along the road:

- Make time for you.

- Make time for healing work, such as meditation, yoga, Reiki, etc.

- Help yourself by changing what isn't good for you (food, alcohol, lack of exercise).

- Practice daily, or regularly.

- Have patience and compassion for yourself.

- Pay attention to your intuition and let it help you make wise decisions about your healing path.

- Let go of the things in your life that are causing you pain, harm, or misfortune.

- Demand space for your growth and awakening.

- Get plenty of good rest and sleep.

- Keep yourself hydrated.

- Accept that change is inevitable and that nothing is permanent.

You can really help yourself open a lot more quickly and pleasantly when you are practicing healthy choices and working with your intuition as you go.

There are certainly times where we will not have space for these exercises or energy clearing methods and that's okay. Life is full of ups and downs, ebbs and flows. There will be plenty of opportunities throughout your chakra awakening experience when you will need to just go with the flow.

- Avoid being rigid and overbearing with your healing experience.

- Avoid engineering impossible goals pertaining to your energy awakening.

- Avoid criticizing your lack of movement forward, especially if you need to just hold space for an important part of your healing work and give time to resettle and transform your energy.

- Avoid living in doubt or fear that you won't be able to do this work and just let it come forward in the right moments for you.

- Avoid boxing yourself into only one way of going through chakra awakening. The experience will be unique to you, so trust your intuition.

Anything that comes up along the way is likely meant to help you resolve some of the physical, mental, and emotional issues that have been a part of your blocked chakra system. It is absolutely normal for there to be strong feelings and emotions surfacing along the way. It is also partly true that things might get a little worse before they start to feel better.

When you are releasing serious illness, trauma, and old wounds from years ago, it can take some time to process and release; but, don't worry! As long as you are taking good care of yourself, trusting your intuition, avoiding things that will set you back, and making space for healing, you will be in good standing and the process will go that much more quickly for you.

Engage with the positive ways you can manage and maintain your chakra awakening experience and prepare to be amazed at how exciting it is to transform through healing your chakras.

You will read through each chakra again, from the root to the crown, to understand each one's imbalances within these categories of self-expression.

Conclusion

Congratulations on finishing the book! If you have read through the entire book, then you are now equipped with the basic knowledge necessary to balance your chakras, free yourself from toxic energy, and experience real healing.

If you are skipping around the book, that's fine too. This book isn't a novel that you are supposed to read once and put aside, it's more like a manual that you should keep on hand so that you know how to deal with any issue that may arise. Reading through the information in this book once is helpful, but you'll need to meditate on the deeper meaning and take concrete steps if you truly want to own this wisdom.

It's all part of the spiritual journey that every one of us is on, whether we know it or not. This book has only scratched the surface of the great mountain of wisdom that has been stored up by countless generations of spiritual seekers.

Now, you are a part of this great chain of humanity that stretches back into the mists of ancient history. Your spiritual potential is unlimited, the only question is how far you are willing to go.

Radiating Energy

The road ahead of you might be long, but if you are open to the universe you will never run out of energy. We live in a universe made of energy. It flows into us and we radiate it out. One of the reasons that we were put on this earth is to play our part in the infinite chain of energy exchange that connects all life and matter in this universe.

It's all about perspective. People without this wide view are often held back from fully embracing practices like yoga and meditation. It is the idea that these are self-centered activities. The thought of spending extended periods of time looking inward can feel like a luxury or an indulgence when the outside world seems to demand our attention at all hours of the day. But the reality is that this whole idea is completely backward. People who are able to look inside of themselves and achieve personal balance are in the best position to bring healing to the entire world.

If you have ever flown on an airplane, then you've seen the song and dance where an airline representative tells you that in case of an emergency, you need to put your own oxygen mask on before you help anyone else. This can seem cruel at first, but it actually speaks to a deep truth. So many people try and sacrifice their own well-being to protect others, only to end up dragging everyone down in the process. If you try to put an oxygen mask on your child, then both of you are likely to end up unconscious. If you try to raise the energy of the world around you without balancing your own energies, then you're just as likely to bring the energy down.

Taking the time to balance your energies and raise your vibration doesn't need to take an eternity. Spending a few minutes, a day in yoga and meditation can create a recognizable uptick in energy. And this energy can be contagious. That's because this world isn't a zero-sum game, where everyone is fighting over a set amount of energy. The truth is that just as each chakra is part of a larger system, the same goes for each person. As each of us balance our own energies, the overall flow of energy increases and the vibration of the species is raised.

One thing you will learn as you discover the deep truths that exist within you and around you is that it's all the same. The systems that exist within you also exist within the planet. The only difference is the scale.

That's the beautiful message of all of this, everything is connected. By healing yourself, you are working to heal the planet. This doesn't mean that you need to feel responsible for the entire world, but it does mean that you don't need to feel like you are helpless in the face of a cold and uncaring world. The truth is that you're a part of a world that is alive and vibrating with the energy of billions of souls.

Today is your chance to heal yourself and heal the world. We're a long way from perfect, but it's like they say, the first step is always the hardest.